THE
BACKCARE BLUEPRINT

End Chronic Back Pain

Without Pills, Shots or Surgery
and Reclaim the Life you Love!

LYNNE ANN PATERSON

THE BACKCARE BLUEPRINT
End Chronic Back Pain Without Pills, Shots or Surgery
and Reclaim the Life You Love!

COVER & INTERIOR LAYOUT: MOLLY SEABROOK DESIGN

I DEDICATE THE BACKCARE BLUEPRINT
TO ALL MY TEACHERS.
I HONOR MY OWN BODY,
THE GREATEST TEACHER,
FOR BEING A FERTILE LABORATORY OF
EXPLORATION, DISCOVERY AND HEALING.
THANK YOU FOR GRACING MY JOURNEY
AND LEADING ME OUT FROM UNDER
THE SHADOW OF PAIN,
BACK TO THE GARDEN OF HEALTH.

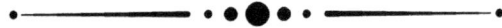

—— · • ● • · ——

THE BODY HEALS WITH PLAY,
THE MIND HEALS WITH LAUGHTER
AND THE SPIRIT HEALS WITH JOY.

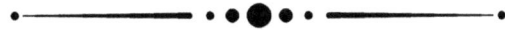

—— · • ● • · ——

TABLE OF CONTENTS

INTRODUCTION

Welcome friend!

You've picked up this book because you, or someone you know, suffers from back pain. Nagging pain! Distracting pain! Serious pain! Chronic pain! More likely than not, you've struggled with back pain for months, years . . . perhaps even decades. In that time, I bet you've popped hundreds of pills in an effort to erase that pain. I presume you've undergone at least one round of physical therapy and/or cortisone shots. Unfortunately, I also know that any respite from back pain is temporary, at best. I'd wager you're hesitant to take stronger medications, like opioids, because you know the risk of addiction outweighs the benefits. And I'd guess you're scared to death of back surgery and wish to avoid that at all costs. It's safe to assume your doctor has run out of suggestions, other than to blame your back pain on aging. You've run out of choices; feeling backed up against a wall with no new options in sight because treatments that once worked are no longer working. Despite these odds, you still yearn to find a way out of back pain—once and for all. You desire a way to restore good health without popping any more pills, getting pricked by another needle, or going under the knife.

Perhaps you've spent a small fortune on complementary treatments like chiropractic care, therapeutic massage, acupuncture, and possibly even energy medicine. And while you certainly enjoyed brief moments without pain, the relief you experienced was only temporary. Merely days after treatment, pain crept into your spine, little by little, and you found yourself right back where you started. Back in pain! What the heck is going on?! This vicious cycle has dragged on for too long, and now you're hanging by a thread at the end of your emotional rope—frustrated, angry, defeated, and exhausted. Just when you'd almost given up all hope, a tiny voice sprang forth from deep within your heart: "There has to be a real solution! I just know it. I've got to keep searching until I find a way out of pain!" And here you are, right now, browsing the self-help book section...and reading this book.

I WANT YOU TO KNOW, I HEAR YOU, LOUD AND CLEAR!

Believe me, I know that you're educated and like to stay informed. I trust you've done your best with the resources and information available to you. I know you are trying your best to cope. By now, you must have realized there's a vital piece of information missing. And if you just knew what that was, or where to find it, you'd feel a whole lot better.

Well, I'm here to tell you something your doctor will probably never say:

There IS a solution! You can heal your body and end back pain yourself. You are in the right place!

WHAT YOU'LL DISCOVER IN THIS BOOK:

The BackCare Blueprint is a natural method of healing that does not require pharmaceutical drugs or medical intervention. It's a system of self-healing that empowers you to sit in the driver's seat of your own healing and regain health. It will help you make the leap from dependency on drugs and doctors to empowered spinal self-care. Thus, it is as boldly unique as it is effective. *The BackCare Blueprint* functions like a roadmap, guiding you back to wholeness. In order to follow a map without getting lost, you need a compass, an experienced guide (me)! familiarity with the terrain, the right gear, a sense of adventure, and a strong belief that it's possible to successfully navigate the path and reach your final destination!

Inside this book, you'll discover specific strategies and proven practices to help you take charge of your spinal health. You'll learn a proven method to mitigate current back pain and prevent future back pain. As you incorporate *The BackCare Blueprint* system into daily life, you'll quickly start to shift out of pain and into a renewed sense of wellbeing and joy! You'll learn to adjust everyday movements like sitting, standing, walking, and bending into powerful allies because this is where you have the most power to transform pain and suffering into freedom and health.

NOT A QUICK FIX:

The BackCare Blueprint is not a "quick fix" self-help book. I won't promise you will heal in seven days or less. It's not another yoga book. You won't learn 108 sun salutations or time-consuming asana sequences. *The BackCare Blueprint* is not a muscle building fitness book. You won't do intense repetitions of core-strengthening crunches or push through an extreme exercise regime. Why? Because they're just not necessary. Most fitness, pain management, and physical therapy programs teach people "what" exercises to practice, but few, if any, teach you "how" to move in a natural way that enhances and speeds healing. My in-depth system will cover exactly "what" you need to do to get out of pain and "how" to do it. In short, where most practitioners aim to fix you, my goal is to guide you to establish the conditions where you can heal yourself.

To be perfectly honest, there is no "quick fix" remedy for chronic back pain. But there IS an effective pathway out of pain. The simple principles of alignment that you'll discover as you read this book, naturally reduce pain and promote healing. My aim is to help you to apply these principles with increased awareness, confidence, and skill as you walk the path towards health.

I will guarantee this: if you follow my recommendations, you can learn to get yourself out of pain and to keep yourself free of pain.

The BackCare Blueprint is not a book for everyone. If you have organic issues such as kidney stones, cysts along the spine, defective surgical hardware (broken pins, protruding screws), systemic toxicity, tumors, etc.—all of which can *cause* back pain—this may not be the right path for you. I have to be honest and admit, I cannot say whether the information provided herein will be of service to you since those organic issues are beyond the scope of my expertise. However, if you are a part of the vast majority of people whose back pain arises from structural misalignment, musculoskeletal imbalance, weak muscles, and poor posture, then I know my method will help you.

WHO AM I TO WRITE THIS BOOK?

In addition to holding several certifications in the healing arts and over 10,000 hours of therapeutic yoga training, I also struggled with chronic sciatic pain for an entire decade. I spent my late twenties and early thirties acting extremely stoic. I slapped on a brave face, pushed through pain, all the while being a miserable wreck on the inside. I didn't sleep much. I cried most nights and grimaced most days. For better or worse, I stubbornly refused to take painkillers. My stubbornness compelled me to find an "all-natural" pathway out of pain, consistent with my "all-natural" approach to life. Ten years later, I finally found the right information and the right guidance. From there, it took me two years to fully heal, naturally. No pills. No shots. No surgery. And no pain! But in order to heal, I had to systematically change the way I used my body both on and off the yoga mat. It took time and diligence, but I healed. What I learned worked so well, I use the same system and practices today, which keep me free from pain tomorrow!

Over the years, while leading public classes, workshops, and working with private clients, I've helped hundreds of people successfully eliminate physical pain from pretty much every part of their body—feet, knees, hips, back, neck, elbows, and wrists. More importantly, I wanted people to heal much faster than I did, so I refined and distilled my methods into a course. In doing so, *the BackCare Blueprint* program and accompanying online video course were born. Now, I can honestly exclaim it's possible for almost anyone to heal back pain within twelve weeks. So please take heart. I feel your pain. I understand exactly where you stand. I've stood there myself.

I promise, wherever you are in your healing journey, *The BackCare Blueprint* will help you decrease pain, reduce suffering, and increase wellbeing, naturally. This system provides new concepts, simple strategies, exceptional tools, effective practices and expert guidance to help you turn pain-inducing habits into pain-reducing proclivities. The methods I lay out in this book will help you eliminate current pain and prevent future pain. I'm truly delighted you've discovered my book. I'm committed to support you on a healing journey to revise your habits, realign your spine and rev up your body's natural healing powers. After all I've been through, after all I've learned, after all I've taught my clients . . . I know what you need to learn to make a successful journey out of pain. This program holds the map and the compass to do so.

My **highest** aim is to imbue you, the reader, with the same knowledge, skills, awareness, and motivation that I used to heal myself; the same system I teach all my students and clients. It is my greatest wish that you take this information and these practices to heart. Use them daily to make significant steps forward in your recovery. May you come to know yourself and your spine more intimately. May you safely return to the activities you love most, with renewed confidence to live life fully. If I could heal . . . if others have healed . . . so can you!

HOW TO USE THIS BOOK:

The BackCare Blueprint provides a starting point for an incredible journey out of pain and back to health. Inside this book, you'll find detailed biomechanical instructions with photos to help you realign the way you sit, stand, walk, bend, twist and breathe.

Part One is the road map. It will help you understand the terrain—the scope of the problem—and why standard medical treatments might be leading you down a dead-end path. It details why your current model of health care fails to serve your best interests and helps you identify general patterns and common habits that contribute to back pain. You'll discover what's missing from the treatment you are currently receiving and you'll start to understand why your back is not getting any better. Without a map, it's easy to stray or get lost. There's no way to get where you want to go without one. If you don't know what's not working and why it's not working, how can you improve? The information in Part One is crucial; that's why it comes first.

Part Two acts like a compass that points you in the direction of healing. It is organized to encourage you to take the first big step on your healing journey: to embrace a new perspective on healing. It will help you see the shortcomings of outdated paradigms and guide you to reorient the way you think about back pain by identifying a personal pattern of pain from one of several common structural misalignments. That pattern becomes your compass needle, indicating when you are in or out of proper alignment. With this knowledge, the optimal posture, or structural blueprint, becomes your North Star. It will show you when you are on course and when you have fallen off course. Your North Star helps you stay on track with your goal of healing back pain yourself.

Part Three is the journey. Armed with personal information from Part One and Part Two, you're ready to start your journey back to health. Here, I introduce specific practices to increase body awareness, improve postural alignment, and harness the power of breath. Ones that you can follow safely at home, at work, or on the go, to relieve back pain. These practices are useful in real time, during your everyday life. I'll show you how to turn common activities like sitting, standing, walking, and bending into strategies for improving your back.

Part Four provides additional resources. During any healing journey, there are times when you get stuck and need extra support. In this section, I cover the use of herbal medicines as a way to support your journey. Herbal medicines are both powerful and effective natural remedies for pain. Some of the herbal allies I list in this section are ones I keep on hand at all times and use on an ongoing basis because they relieve pain without any negative side effects.

If you still need extra support, check out the online video companion course for *The BackCare Blueprint* book. It contains several dozen short practice videos (between 3–15 minutes in length) that demonstrate "how" to apply sound, biomechanical alignment principles in everyday poses—the same ones I present in this book. These simple exercises and short sequences will make your back feel better quickly. If you need individual help, please reach out to me in person. You'll find my contact information in the resource section at the end of this book.

Remember—to embed new habits of movement, breath and posture takes time and commitment until they become familiar and automatic. But managing your own posture and habits is still one of the most effective ways (dare I say THE most effective way) to take charge of your own health, ditch the meds, and finally learn to heal yourself from chronic back pain.

THE BOTTOM LINE IS THIS:

I want you to know that while chronic pain can ruin a life, it does NOT have to ruin yours! You've got more life to live, don't you want to enjoy the ride? More importantly, you've got boat loads to lose—your quality and your love of life—if you don't resolve your chronic back pain soon. Chronic back pain is your wake-up call. Don't ignore it. Chronic pain asks you to reexamine your daily lifestyle and habits and to view this issue as a monumental opportunity to reorient your direction. Perhaps this is why you were drawn to my book. The information, tips and practices provided in *The BackCare Blueprint* will help you reclaim your vitality and enjoyment of life. Without realizing it, you've just taken the most important step: you've finally discovered a method of self-healing that will actually help you. So now it's time to learn what you can do to free yourself from pain.

Read on . . . I've got your back!

Lynne

PART ONE

THE NOT-SO-SILENT EPIDEMIC

There comes a time in everyone's life when one feels compelled to take matters into their own hands. Most often the urgency to act arises when one's own self, family, community, or country are at risk of harm or in danger. With the myriad of ways that modern medicine has fallen short of curing chronic back pain in those who suffer, a great many people seek a different pathway forward. Perhaps you feel that urgency, too, because you've suffered long enough. In Part One, we'll peel back the veil and look at the hard facts about what has prevented you from healing chronic back pain.

CHAPTER 1

THE PAINFUL TRUTH ABOUT CHRONIC BACK PAIN

"When you get to the end of your rope, tie a knot and hang on."

— *Theodore Roosevelt*

According to WebMD, over 540 million people worldwide, 10% of the global population, suffer from back pain. In America alone, over 86 million hard-working people currently endure back pain. And while standard medical treatments—pills, shots, physical therapy and surgery—can help people with acute spinal injuries, more often than not, these treatments fail to cure those suffering with chronic back pain. In many cases, allopathic medicine is simply not equipped to address chronic back pain, much less fix it. Let's find out why.

Pharmaceutical painkillers mask pain, instead of harnessing pain to investigate the root cause of one's discomfort. Cortisone shots, a common treatment for back pain, are reported to provide temporary relief only 50% of the time. The same results are seen with physical therapy—only half of people in physical therapy find relief, the other half do not. The same percentage holds true for my clients.

Often, standard treatments like back surgery end up causing more pain. It's been reported that spinal surgery provides permanent pain relief in only .002% patients. With such a terribly low (basically zero) success rate, why would anyone opt for a high-risk intervention? As you may realize, the modern western health care system is broken. Many doctors prescribe standard treatments rather than spend extra time to uncover and address the root cause of chronic back pain. It's not entirely their fault, as the health insurance system works against both doctors and patients by limiting the length of a typical office visit. And working one's way through the medical system can take months, even years.

Over the past twenty years, the occurrence of back pain has been on a steady rise, and there is no sign of it slowing. An average 8 out of 10 adults will struggle with back pain at some time in their life. More women (30%) will suffer with lower back pain than men (25%). Routinely, men perform harder physical labor tasks than women, so wouldn't we expect the percentage of men with lower back pain to be higher than women? If not from physical labor or physical injury, what's the source of chronic back pain for women? More men report back injury at work than their female co-workers. Why is that? What's going on? Do women need help, but avoid asking for it? Or are they less capable of speaking up on their own behalf? It appears that many men muscle through pain, while many women struggle in silence. And you? How are you braving back pain or pushing through it?

Back pain affects people in every aspect of their lives by making simple daily tasks a challenge. Pain limits the ability to move and reduces the desire to exercise. Why, chronic back pain even impairs sleep. In America, over $50 billion dollars are spent on back pain treatment each year, and yet the number of people with persistent back pain continues to rise. The impact of this not-so-silent epidemic spreads into all aspects of life. Currently over $100 billion dollars are accrued indirectly as lost wages, decreased productivity, insurance and legal fees. You'd think by throwing huge amounts of money at a problem we'd find a solution! But that is not what is happening. The problem is getting worse! More people are in more pain today, rather than in less pain. Why is this?

There's a huge gap between scientific knowledge and common medical practice. Between triage, prevention, and treatment. Doctors, physical therapists, and chiropractors are trained to treat symptoms and syndromes, but not to educate their patients to prevent pain and illness. Unfortunately for us, it's far more lucrative to manage pain than it is to cure pain. The status quo medical system is designed to keep patients on the hook, coming back for an endless string of tests, treatments, adjustments or surgery. As Dr. Glenn Melnick, Ph.D., and Professor of Health Care Finance at USC, said: "Healthcare is now so dysfunctional that I sometimes think the only solution is to blow the whole thing up."

CONCLUSION

Obviously, the current western medical model of health needs a total makeover, and so do you! What's needed most is a major shift from managing back pain to the promotion of self-healing and prevention. And that's exactly what you'll get from reading this book. My aim is to educate you to heal your current back pain, prevent future back pain, and provide viable strategies to get out of pain, should your back pain ever return. So rather than blow up the entire system, let's make a distinction between the types of issues you can address yourself and those which might require medical intervention. We'll begin by looking at four modern postural problems.

> "
>
> *The current western medical model of health needs a total makeover, and so do you!*

CHAPTER 2

21ST CENTURY SYNDROMES

"Pain is inevitable, suffering is optional." — *Buddhist Proverb*

In the last few decades, four new epidemics—what I call "21st century syndromes"—have appeared within the general populace. They are the direct result of an increasingly sedentary lifestyle coupled with excessive use of technology, poor structural alignment, negative mindset, and lackluster breathing. While it's important to take responsibility for your own health, it's equally important to acknowledge the likelihood that you've been raised in a culture of healthcare which robs you of personal power. One that places the power to heal in the hands of authorities outside yourself and emphasizes the outdated and disempowering belief that you cannot heal yourself.

The following four syndromes—sitter's disease, weak butt syndrome, slouchy shoulder, and text neck—are finally gaining recognition as issues that cause real physiological illness. These new postural patterns have become completely ingrained in the body due to sedentary lifestyles and the chronic use of technology. Many people are not even aware that the posture may be at the root of their back pain. But knowledge is power! When you become aware of the structural causes of back pain, you can take positive actions to remedy them—yourself.

> *When you become aware of the structural causes of back pain, you can take positive actions to remedy them—yourself.*

"SITTER'S DISEASE"

Did you know the most frequent issue people complain about to their doctor is lower back pain? Or that more than half of ALL office workers (54%) struggle with back pain? Lower back pain is the number one reason why people visit their doctor or chiropractor. So, what causes this upward trending syndrome?

It's a well-known fact that Americans sit, on average, eleven hours every day. Prolonged sitting—anything over six hours—is now considered a serious health risk. Sitting is considered THE new smoking! A 2011 research study revealed that prolonged sitting increases the risk of more than thirty-four chronic diseases, including diabetes, obesity, cardiovascular disease, and cancer. In fact, people who sit twelve to fifteen hours each day and offset sitting by daily exercise have the same health risks as people who do not exercise at all. Seriously! Even worse, prolonged sitting nearly doubles the risk of an early death. That's a terrifying statistic. This massive trend has led to a new medical term: "sitter's disease."

Currently 40% of all people who suffer with back pain see a doctor and chiropractor equally. In addition, 20% seek out a spinal health specialist. Even with excellent medical care, ONLY one out of ten patients ever finds out the root cause of their back pain. That means a whopping nine out of ten patients NEVER discover what caused their pain in the first place. If you don't know what caused pain and injury, how can you avoid pain? How can you heal it? Why aren't more doctors looking for the cause? And what do the 60% of people who never see a doctor do about their back pain? Do they suffer in silence? Pop more painkillers and return to work? What about you? How many hours a day do you sit, slumping at a desk, computer, or car? What risks do you face and what are you doing to alleviate the pain?

"WEAK BUTT" SYNDROME

As a direct result of a sedentary lifestyle—sitting at a desk staring into your computer or sitting at home on the couch watching TV—another big problem has appeared. This one is called the "weak butt" syndrome. When you sit more than you move, every system in your body loses function and your body grows weaker. Prolonged sitting constantly weakens core muscles which become unable to hold the spine in an optimal upright aligned position. When your core (which includes the muscles of the pelvis, hips, hamstrings, abdominals and lower back) lack strength, the spine is negatively affected. Without proper support of an integrated core, the spinal muscles become weak, the vertebrae become misaligned, and unnatural pressure is put on the disks and nerves. In this way, structural misalignment becomes a prime source of back pain. While weak butt syndrome and sitter's disease are related, it's possible to have one without the other. Of course, getting up and walking around once an hour for several minutes can help, but did you know there are things you can do while sitting that can help relieve and prevent pain? No? Well, I'll teach you how to counter "weak butt" syndrome in Part Three.

"SLOUCHY SHOULDER" AND "TEXT NECK" SYNDROMES

Slouchy shoulder and text neck syndromes are also modern problems resulting from the prolonged habit of dropping the head, neck and shoulders while staring down at a computer, keyboard, phone, any electronic screen, or even at print material. Slouchy shoulder syndrome happens when you slouch your upper body. The arms hang down from the shoulder sockets pulling the shoulder girdle away from the head. This position strains the muscles of the neck, shoulders and upper back. This is a very common habit whether you work at a desk or stare at a screen, as it's impossible to keep the spine and head upright and only slouch the shoulders. Text neck (or tech neck) occurs from the use of hand-held devices, where the user stands or sits up straight but drops only the head forward and down, instead of lifting the device up to eye level. It's very common to have both slouchy shoulders AND text neck because the weight of the head dropping down pulls the shoulder girdle forward and arms down, too.

In either case, in order to "stay connected" to others at work, school, or on social media, people disconnect from their body and misalign their spine. Tilting your head forward and down pulls the entire spine out of alignment. The weight of the skull puts up to sixty pounds of pressure into the delicate vertebrae of the neck. A chronically forward-rounded position over stretches the neck and upper back muscles, which cry out in pain for relief. Both slouchy shoulder syndrome and text neck are issues of misuse, underuse, and overuse. I've seen many older people who can barely stand upright because these poor postural habits have become completely embedded in their body. Don't let that happen to you! Get up and walk around with your eyes looking forward—not down—each hour to help offset those harmful positions. In Part Three, I'll teach you how to counter these 21st century syndromes with simple and effective alignment techniques.

Right now, write down which syndrome is likely your main issue:

_____

_____

_____

STRUCTURAL MISALIGNMENT

Each of the above four "21st century syndromes" is a direct result of structural misalignment.

A structural misalignment results from bones that shift out of natural alignment because the muscles, tendons, ligaments and fascia that should support and hold

> **Seventy-five percent of ALL back pain arises from a misaligned body!**

them in place are either too weak to hold the spine in proper position or so tight they pull the vertebrae out of alignment. Prolonged sitting and improper posture can adversely affect these tissues (and the organs) by continuously putting stress on the spinal vertebrae, discs and nerves. Physical misalignment impairs the movement of blood, lymph and craniosacral fluid and decreases your ability to breathe deeply. When the body's 'waters of life' are restricted, vitality is lost. When breath is constricted or diminished, one's whole health is compromised. I'll expand these ideas in Part Two, but for now it's imperative to acknowledge a widely accepted fact:

Seventy-five percent of ALL back pain arises from structural misalignment.

Yes, I repeat:

Seventy-five percent of ALL back pain arises from a misaligned body!

In my opinion, structural misalignment is the cause of many common spinal issues from which back pain arises, including:

1. **Herniated disc (bulging or ruptured)**—where the nucleus of the spinal disc leaks through cracks (called annular fissures) of the outer layer of the disc putting pressure on the nerves of the spinal canal.

2. **Compression of vertebrae**—which can cause degeneration of the bones and damage to the nerves and discs, as well as inflaming the tissues.

3. **Arthritis or facet joint disease**—where the spinal processes and facet joints of the vertebrae become inflamed and irritated.

4. **Spinal curvatures**—including scoliosis ("S" or "C" curves), kyphosis (excess upper back curve), lordosis (excess lower back curve), flat back (no curve) or reversed curve.

5. **Sacro-iliac joint pain**—caused by external torsion of the leg, which can displace the ilium (pelvic) bone putting pressure into the SI joint.

6. **Slipped vertebrae** (spondylolisthesis)—where one vertebra slips forward and out of alignment with the vertebrae above and below it, putting pressure on the disc and nerves.

7. **Sciatica**—often caused by a herniated disc or misaligned vertebra in the lumbar spine (L1-L5) that puts pressure on the sciatic nerve. Sciatic pain radiates from the lower back, down through the buttock, back of the thigh, and into the calf or foot.

8. **Piriformis Syndrome** — a spasm in the piriformis muscle of the buttock can irritate the sciatic nerve, causing pain, numbness or tingling that radiate down the back of the leg, into the calf or foot. This sensation is similar to that of sciatic pain.

As you can see, structural misalignment—more commonly known as 'poor posture'—is at the root of much back pain. However, correcting poor posture is more sophisticated than simply sitting, or standing up straight, or pulling in your stomach. A delicate balance between opposing muscles must be established in order to correct structural misalignment while safeguarding the joints, vertebrae, and discs of the spine.

Every person—yourself included—has a unique pattern of misalignment which causes certain parts of the back to hurt or specific types of issues to arise. And while this may sound complex, I assure you anyone can learn to properly correct poor postural patterns, realign their spine, and alleviate most or all chronic back pain. You'll discover exactly how to do so as you read Part Three.

First, let's look at three contributing issues.

UNDERUSE, OVERUSE, MISUSE

Over the years, I've noticed the habits of my clients with chronic back pain fall into one of three categories: underuse, misuse, or overuse.

Underuse

Sitter's disease and weak butt syndrome are both perfect examples of *underuse*. In a sedentary culture, it's very common that the core muscles of the body weaken over time from lack of use. When this occurs, the core muscles, which include the abdominals, buttocks, hamstrings and lower back, cannot properly support the skeleton, and it sags out of alignment. This misalignment puts excess gravitational pressure into the joints, discs, nerves and soft tissues of the spine and pelvis. That pressure can, and often does, cause a tremendous amount of pain. Excess pressure can also result in spinal compression, degenerative disc disease, herniated discs, and nerve impingement. Underuse also occurs with slouchy shoulder and text neck syndromes, but in this case, it's the muscles of the middle and upper back and neck that weaken from constant misalignment, while the muscles of the front of the chest tighten. Of course, you might think the remedy for all four syndromes is simply to exercise more often (or at all), and while I agree, exercise done with poor alignment often causes more physical pain or can result in injury.

Overuse

Overuse shows up as the slow wear 'n tear from years of moving the body with improper alignment and imbalanced muscle tone. Overuse results from ignoring the body's signs of fatigue and its need for rest. Unfortunately, too many people force themselves to work past their body's limit, increasing the risk of injury. Pushing past one's physical limits with a structural misalignment can potentially result in minor injury, such muscle strain, sprain, or micro-tears. Pain arises—not from a sudden tweak or dramatic physical injury, as in misuse—but from repeating misaligned movement again and again.

I know many carpenters who tell me how broken their body feels after years of physical labor "all in the name of a good day's work." Now they're paying the price in the currency of chronic pain for being harsh on their bodies for many decades. Overuse of certain muscles implies underuse of others, so it's important to build up weak muscles without over-developing already strong muscles. In the end, it's a balanced use of muscular action that facilitates healing.

Misuse

When the body is used incorrectly over time or moved suddenly without proper alignment, the risk of injury skyrockets. A perfect and common example of misuse is rounding the back while bending over to pick something up. This action puts undue stress on the muscles, ligaments, tendons, and joints of the spine. Reaching suddenly for something in the back seat of the car is another common way people tweak their back. Lifting and carrying objects heavier than what your muscle strength can tolerate may cause injury. When the body is constantly misused and injured, it gets weaker . . . and before you know it, you've crossed a breaking point.

As a result, you could cause more than minor damage to your tissues. You might tear a tendon or muscle, overstretch a ligament, pull a vertebra out of alignment, herniate a disc, or damage a nerve, all of which can result in more and possibly excruciating pain!

Since most people live in a crazy, busy culture where the demands on their time are constantly under siege, the pressure to get things done quickly is relentless. It's a do more, get more done mentality. When this is your primary way of life, it's almost impossible to give your body the rest it needs when it needs it, or to move slowly and mindfully so you can avoid harm. To misuse your body is to risk injury! Get the idea?

While most people underuse, overuse, or misuse their body in some way at some time in their life, not every person ends up with chronic back pain. For those who

> *A perfect template or blueprint for the human body already exists— one where the body is designed to move expressively, freely, and without pain.*

do, until you understand what **you** do to cause yourself pain and address that cause, you may continue to endure pain no matter how many pills you pop, or how often you receive cortisone shots, physical therapy, chiropractic adjustments, massage treatments, or acupuncture sessions. Why? Because you're still operating from an outdated modality of healthcare that does not correct the root cause.

THE BOTTOM LINE

The good news is that a perfect template or blueprint for the human body already exists—one where the body is designed to move expressively, freely, and without pain. The way to remedy chronic back pain caused by structural misalignment and create natural, joyful movement is the science of biomechanics. The basic principles of biomechanics—how your body is designed to move—are not hard to master. The steps to rebalance your posture and master simple biomechanical alignment is what I offer in *The BackCare Blueprint* and accompanying video course. Once you understand your habit of underuse, overuse, or misuse, you can learn to identify and adjust your particular pattern of misalignment to reestablish the original blueprint. When you do, you'll be well on your way to reducing pain and healing your back, because a body in balance can and will heal. I hope you're excited to discover the healing method you were seeking!

CHAPTER 3
A PAINFUL STATE OF AFFAIRS

"All the world is full of suffering. It is also full of overcoming." — *Helen Keller*

Remember as a child, how you played with such joyful abandon? And how over time, as you grew up and went to work, your physical movements became less varied, less expressive? Now you find yourself stuck at a desk, with a spine so stiff that your limited range of motion has put a damper on the fun you'd otherwise be having. Seriously, ignoring these 21st century syndromes and neglecting to address underuse, overuse, or misuse can lead to some serious problems.

You may have heard that 90% of all people who tweak their back heal naturally within five to six weeks. Or that back pain will go away with simple rest, if you take time to rest. But did you know that 8% of people (68 million) with back pain experience a resurgence of back pain within two years of the first incident? After that, back pain occurs more frequently, not less. Why is this?

Reinjury and Recurrent Pain

Admittedly, once you've hurt your back, you're at greater risk of reinjury. The damaged tissues become weaker and more susceptible to injury unless you do something to radically retrain your habits. Every time you reinjure your back, back pain returns. Pain is typically the first sign people notice that indicates something has gone wrong—again! But pain is actually the second thing that happens. And it happens after each injury. Because of repeated injury—even minor injury—the body never quite fully heals. Can you see how prolonged pain indicates that injured tissue has not fully healed, and that same tissue is repetitively reinjured?

Over time, you get stuck in a cycle of partial healing: as your body starts to improve, pain goes away; when you reinjure yourself, back pain returns. You're dealing with cyclical pain, not constant pain. Some days you feel great, other times you pop pills to get through the day. This "on and off" pain which occurs repeatedly and often over time is called "recurrent" pain. It is caused by repeated injury (reinjury). It's important to note that both reinjury and recurrent pain are caused by habitual patterns of misuse, overuse or underuse—all of which result from incorrect patterns of movement and posture that are constantly misaligned. (Remember, 75% of all back pain is from a structural issue.)

If you've read this far, it's very likely that you suffer from recurrent back pain. Most of my therapeutic yoga clients endured recurrent back pain for more than five years before seeking my help. Many of my clients carried back pain around for over twenty years, some for over thirty years.

During the first few years of my battle with sciatica, I experienced recurrent pain in my lower back and right leg. Without realizing, every time I practiced deep forward bends or stretched my legs straight, I re-tore my hamstrings. I failed to recognize the root problem: my own habitual patterns of misuse, overuse, and misalignment. In short, I had no idea how to stretch my hamstrings safely without constantly damaging them. Unfortunately, this gross lack of knowledge and understanding in my twenties morphed into a pattern of reinjury where I suddenly found myself with back and leg pain all the time! I needed to understand what I was doing wrong so I could change the pattern, heal the tissues, and stop the pain.

Habitual Misalignment & Repetitive Trauma:

It's important to understand that repeated underuse, overuse, or misuse of the body coupled with habitual misalignment and cyclic reinjury are what prevent you from fully healing. These are also the reasons why recurrent back pain so stubbornly refuses to abate. Prolonged habitual misalignment with poor muscle tone puts you at constant risk of reinjuring yourself with greater frequency. Any injury causes trauma

> "
> *Over time, you get stuck in a cycle of partial healing: as your body starts to improve, pain goes away; when you reinjure yourself, back pain returns.*

to the tissues of your body, but frequently repeated reinjury causes "repetitive trauma." With repetitive trauma, the parts of your body originally damaged suffer trauma over and over again. The level of intensity caused by this constant trauma is experienced on multiple levels—physical, emotional and mental, simultaneously. In many cases, this sustained discomfort is enough to drive anyone to pop painkillers or have a drink to numb the extreme sensation. If the pattern of misalignment is not remedied, the body can become locked in a cycle of reinjury and repetitive trauma from which the cycle of chronic pain arises.

Do you now understand which pattern—misuse, underuse, overuse, reinjury or repetitive trauma negatively affects you and makes your back hurt?

If so, jot the pattern down here:

_____

_____

_____

Now I have to state clearly that reinjury and repetitive trauma cannot be healed by doing the same movements in the same way!

They can only be healed by doing the same movements differently. Or by doing different movements correctly. Obviously, the old pattern of how you carry your body has to change. Breaking the cycle of repetitive trauma is two-fold; first, you need to learn what you are currently doing that causes reinjury and repetitive trauma, and second, you must learn how to break that cycle by forming new postural habits and healthier movement patterns. For some people, all that's needed are a

> *If the pattern of misalignment is not remedied, the body can become locked in a cycle of reinjury and repetitive trauma from which the cycle of chronic pain arises.*

few simple postural tweaks. For others, a total postural makeover is required. Either way, to transform poor habits of underuse, overuse, or misuse into healthy aligned movement will eventually create a pain-free experience.

It took me decades to realize that I had been causing reinjury and repetitive trauma for years, which led to the onset of chronic pain. And because I had to piece my healing together by myself, it took two years to finally break out of that chronic pain cycle and fully heal.

The great news is this:

As you learn to use your body more intelligently, with the help of the alignment techniques in Part Three, you can resolve issues of misuse, overuse, and underuse. You can end the cycle of repetitive trauma and chronic pain once-and-for-all. And if you dedicate yourself to this exploration it won't take you years, or decades, to heal. Now that you know which pattern—misuse, underuse, overuse, reinjury or repetitive trauma is dogging you, let's look at the vicious cycle of chronic pain.

THE CYCLE OF CHRONIC PAIN:

Repeated reinjury causes both recurrent pain and repetitive trauma. From here, it's easy to descend into a chronic pain pattern. Chronic pain is any pain that consistently persists, unabated, for three months or longer. Medically speaking, "chronic" is a condition or experience that is constant, perpetual, and persists for such a long time it becomes difficult to eradicate. According to conventional thinking, chronic pain outlasts the usual healing period and becomes progressively worse over time because it is so difficult to resolve. Some doctors and their patients consider chronic pain to be incurable. But I disagree.

In this chronic pain model, tissue damage from an injury is at the epicenter. When a physical injury occurs, pain is the first physical sensation to arise. The normalcy you enjoyed before an injury is disturbed by the sensation of pain. Here, the central nervous system sends disruptive signals to your mind and heart, affecting your thoughts and emotions. Then, suffering at the physical level simultaneously ripples out into the mental and emotional levels.

When suffering is prolonged, the quality of one's thoughts and emotions take a turn for the worse. You might feel disheartened, or worse, become depressed because you have not fully healed. You might start believing that you'll never heal. These "negative" thoughts send messages to the body that actually increase pain, prolong injury, and interfere with healing.

If the injury does not heal in an appropriate amount of time, not only is suffering prolonged, but dramatic changes can occur in one's behavior. Many people become afraid to do activities they once loved for fear of experiencing more pain. And so, they decide to forego that activity. Over time with less and less activity, they fall further out of shape. The muscles that should hold the spine in position become weaker and pain becomes stronger.

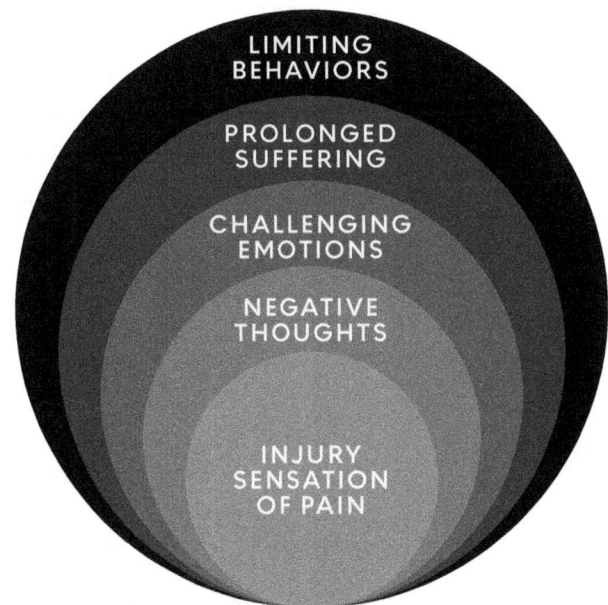

LIMITING BEHAVIORS

PROLONGED SUFFERING

CHALLENGING EMOTIONS

NEGATIVE THOUGHTS

INJURY SENSATION OF PAIN

CHRONIC PAIN MODEL

When chronic pain debilitates your quality of life on all these levels you become a different person. The consequences of not being proactive, not taking steps to end repeated injury and repetitive trauma, are enormous. As soon as you stop living life as accustomed, the relationship with people around you also changes, typically, for the worse. All of these changes—physical, emotional, and mental—exacerbate the original pain, and soon life plummets into a downward spiral where you become stuck in the cycle of chronic pain.

Now, everyone has stubbed a toe, sprained an ankle, cut a finger, and experienced bumps and bruises. Some have broken a bone. Every injury goes through the same steps of healing from the moment of impact to the return of wholeness. Acute pain experienced at the time of injury normally diminishes as healing progresses. That is to say—pain and swelling go down as healing occurs. We declare healing is complete when we no longer experience pain.

But if you are one of the 86 million Americans who currently suffer with chronic pain, this natural healing cycle has been interrupted; it never comes to an end. You're stuck with a recurring pattern of reinjury from which you never fully heal. You'd expect a particular injury to heal over a specific length of time, depending on the type of injury and the level of one's health at the time of injury, but when the healing cycle does not proceed according to Nature, or when it is interrupted by reinjury, pain does not resolve. Instead, it lingers for months, years, even decades. Here, the pattern of chronic pain becomes established in your system.

So, what's at the root of chronic pain?

To understand the cause, let's look at a different definition, one that reveals an extremely important point: **chronic 'anything' is habitual. H-A-B-I-T-U-A-L.** Typically, we associate "chronic" with something we don't wish to experience—like constant pain—but it is imperative that we make the connection between chronic pain and habitually bad habits. To say it another way: chronically poor postural habits *cause* chronic back pain! This can be wonderfully eye-opening news! Why? Because any habitual pattern can be remedied with a sincere desire to change, mindful attention, and dedicated practice.

The key to break the cycle is to identify the underlying postural habit at the root of your reinjury/recurrent pain/repetitive trauma pattern. Address this primary habit according to the natural blueprint of the human body, and you can stop reinjuring and retraumatizing yourself long enough to allow the damaged tissue to heal. When you do, chronic pain will finally end. Hallelujah!!

Now, not every person with back pain falls down into a chronic pain blackhole. Some people have a significant structural misalignment but never experience back pain. Some have a high tolerance level and aren't bothered by pain. But many people put up with low-grade pain for years, even decades, because they've been told they cannot heal, or they believe they'll never heal. And many folks are unmotivated to make changes because they cannot see the direct connection between chronic habits and chronic pain. They don't understand how they might be creating more pain by what they do or by what they avoid.

If you're thinking, "I'm exhausted from living with pain, pain, pain! I'm sick of taking pills. Cortisone shots and physical therapy didn't help. I've done everything my doctors recommended, but I definitely don't want surgery! I've spent a small fortune out-of-pocket for weekly chiropractic, massage and acupuncture sessions . . . and my back still aches. How the heck did I plummet down from good health then get stuck in a chronic cycle of back pain? What should I do now? Where do I start?" I understand your frustration. You're stuck in a cycle of recurrent back pain and/or repetitive trauma, spinning your wheels trying to find a way out. Your best intentions

> *Chronically poor postural habits cause chronic back pain!*

37

and efforts have not paid off. You certainly wouldn't be reading this book if any of the treatments you tried provided a permanent solution and put an end to chronic back pain!

This conundrum is not of your making!! It's not your fault!

Everyone in our culture lacks preventative health education because there's little monetary funding for it. But that's only part of the problem, which I'll speak more about in the next chapter. The other half of the problem is that we've all grown up deferring our authority to doctors and giving our power away to the healthcare system. We must reclaim the personal power and knowledge to heal ourselves.

If you truly desire to end chronic back pain, please ask yourself: *am I willing to make the necessary changes to my patterns to avoid becoming one of the 65 million Americans and 577 million people worldwide enslaved by back pain? Am I willing to shift my habits, posture, and remedy issues of underuse, overuse and misuse? Am I interested to discover how I contribute to my own back pain and learn how to stop injuring myself?*

If you said "yes" to even one of these questions, you're in the right place. The book you're holding is your best next step. The time for healing is here.

In the next chapter, I'll show you why and discuss what I believe to be the five most crucial missing links that contribute to these patterns and set you up for failure. Without knowing what's missing, you can't figure out what to do or how to proceed.

CHAPTER 4

THE FIVE MISSING LINKS

"Often it isn't the initiating trauma or injury that creates seemingly insurmountable pain, but the lack of support thereafter." — Unknown

From where I stand, outside of the allopathic medical paradigm, I've noticed there are five missing links within the modern American health care system. Each broken link in the chain of health blocks the path forward and reduces your chances of healing chronic back pain.

1. MISSING: A LACK OF KNOWLEDGE ON THE HUMAN BODY

You are so much more than a physical body, but western medicine only treats physical symptoms, often ignoring the root cause of pain. In order to heal chronic back pain, it's essential that you are treated as a living physical and spiritual being. You are not a car whose parts are easily replaced. The human blueprint of your physical body is not separate from your mind, emotions, breath, or Spirit—it contains them all. You are never separate, nor will you ever be separate. *The BackCare Blueprint* program begins to address misalignment in the physical, mental and breath bodies with specific practices to bring the whole system back into balance.

The instructions in Part Three are given in detail, and if you follow them you will see improvement. More than half of my clients heal with only the information presented in *The BackCare Blueprint* book. Only a few clients have required support that goes beyond the physical body because their issues were rooted in deeper mental, emotional or spiritual layers.

> *The human blueprint of your physical body is not separate from your mind, emotions, breath, or Spirit — it contains them all.*

2. MISSING: A LACK OF PATIENT EDUCATION

While most doctors and healthcare practitioners treat their patients, they seldom educate patients on how to better care for themselves. Perhaps they lack the training and knowledge to do so, or perhaps they want to keep you tethered to the western medical system, forever. Or maybe it's both. I cannot say which is true for your doctor because both skillful and negligent healthcare workers exist. Since doctors mainly prescribe pharmaceuticals and surgeons perform operations for a living, it's fair to say these are the only solutions allopathic doctors will offer you. If you're suffering with chronic back pain, it's high time to educate yourself about your body. *The BackCare Blueprint* program will help you do just that.

3. MISSING: A LACK OF PATIENT PARTICIPATION

If you are not an active participant in your own healing, how do you think you will ever improve? A lack of participation is not completely your fault. Over the last century, since the advent of modern medicine, we've been conditioned (from birth to burial) to seek answers and healing from doctors and authority figures outside ourselves and to obey them without question. I hope the information provided here will inspire and motivate you to become an active participant in your own healing journey. It is the most important step missing from modern healthcare. Use the tools and tips provided within to become the driver of your own health and have the courage to become your own authority.

4. MISSING: A LACK OF ONGOING SUPPORT

What happens between doctor visits or chiropractic appointments? More likely than not, you resort to the same old habits that got you into this mess in the first place. This is not your fault, either. The modern health care system is not structured to help you prevent illness or to make lasting changes. While your doctor may tell you what you need to do, like lose weight, he or she does not and cannot support you to make those necessary changes. Doctors are much too busy. You may be advised on what changes to make, but you won't receive the guidance or support to make them. You're left on your own!

Without ongoing support between appointments or sessions to keep you motivated and on track, it's nearly impossible to make and sustain effective change by yourself. At the end of the book, you'll find resources including information about my online video course and 1:1 coaching program, both designed to provide additional support, help you stay the course, and maximize your healing journey.

5. MISSING: A LACK OF ACCOUNTABILITY

A lack of accountability goes hand-in-hand with a lack of ongoing support. There is a huge, missed opportunity to transfer responsibility for health and wellness from provider to patient. Since you've been trained to rely on others to make you healthy, it can be a long road to become fully accountable for your habits, actions, thoughts, and feelings. But it can be done!

An expert guide is someone like me, designated to help you stay on track, press through challenging moments, and celebrate breakthroughs and successes. When you follow the practices in *The BackCare Blueprint*, you will make steady progress. The more accountable you are to yourself, the faster you'll get out of pain. I promise. When you're in need of extra support or guidance, please reach out to me.

It is at this point I'm compelled to pause and tell you about Mark. Mark was the CEO of a local non-profit and a lifelong meditator. By the time we met, he'd already spent thirty

> *After eight weeks...all the pain of the past thirty years vanished.*

years trying to resolve chronic back pain. Mark told me he'd "seen everyone and tried everything." His doctor ran a battery of tests, but never found anything wrong. In fact, his doctor actually told Mark that the back pain he experienced was a natural part of aging he'd have to live with. But Mark did not give up. He saw all the best chiropractors, acupuncturists, massage therapists, and energy healers in the area. After these sessions, he'd feel great for a few days, but the pain always returned. When he'd exhausted his search without finding permanent relief, he sought me out, figuring he had nothing to lose by trying something different. Meeting with me was his last resort, his "Hail Mary" pass.

"With all the knowledgeable and skillful practitioners you've seen, didn't anyone teach you how to help yourself?" I asked him. "No," he replied. "Well, you're in the right place," I said. "I know exactly how to help you. I will teach you how to heal yourself." And that began a three-month collaborative journey where I'd observe Mark's patterns of movement and then educate him to stand, sit, walk, bend, and twist properly, without any pain at all. After eight weeks, he experienced a huge breakthrough and all the pain of the past thirty years vanished. During the final weeks of his program, we worked to instill new attitudes, beliefs, patterns, and maintain good posture until finally Mark knew exactly what and how to keep himself out of pain. Perhaps, after reading Mark's story, you see my point! Although Mark received excellent care from very skillful practitioners, he still lacked the necessary education, support, accountability and motivation to end his chronic back pain, once and for all, and on his own.

Now, before you read further, take a moment to jot down—in order of priority—which link or links are missing from your current health care treatment plan and why?

_____

_____

_____

_____

_____

_____

_____

_____

_____

_____

PATIENT EDUCATION

PATIENT PARTICIPATION

HUMAN BLUEPRINT

ONGOING SUPPORT

ACCOUNTABILITY

FIVE MISSING LINKS

DIAGNOSIS

Before we proceed, I must mention other causes of persistent back pain, since approximately 25% of all people with back pain do not have a problematic structural misalignment. Back pain can also be caused by congenital malformation, advanced osteoporosis, cysts, benign or malignant tumors, toxicity, pathogens, infection, abscess, or Ankylosing Spondylitis (AS), a rare type of arthritis. Inflammation, if not from an acute injury, or AS, can arise from nutritional imbalances or gut issues. It's possible there could be a disruption in your body's electromagnetic energy field, an imbalance in biochemistry, a short circuit in the nervous system, a sleep disorder, or an unresolved trauma that adds emotional and psychological stress (and pain!) to your suffering.

Since the causes of back pain are many, what could also be missing from your approach is a professional medical diagnosis. While typical allopathic medical treatments of pills, shots, and surgeries often fall short in resolving chronic back pain, I do believe a medical diagnosis can provide very useful information. It's an important starting point, if you've had pain for more than several months, especially if you've been popping meds, putting on a brave face, and pushing through pain.

The four main diagnostic tools used to examine the cervical spine (neck), thoracic spine (middle back), and lumbar spine (lower back) are:

1. X-rays

X-rays provide an assessment of the curvature alignment of the bones of the spine, including vertebral body fracture (from an injury), scoliosis and kyphosis (curvatures of the spine), spondylolisthesis (spinal dislocation), and other abnormalities such as bone spurs, disc space narrowing (spinal stenosis), and degeneration. X-rays indicate if you're among the 75% of people with structural issues.

2. MRI's

MRIs provide detailed assessment of the bones, soft tissues and organs. They can reveal damage to the spinal cord, nerves, and discs. MRIs will show a herniated disc, narrowing of the spinal canal (spinal stenosis), damage to the spinal cord, nerves and nerve endings, and even spinal compression. They can also indicate injury or inflammation of the muscles, tendons and ligaments. An MRI can indicate if you're one of the 25% of people whose pain is from something other than structural misalignment.

3. CT (CAT) Scan

CT Scan is a specialized x-ray that provides more detailed images than a regular x-ray. These tests yield information about soft tissue and bones. They can reveal complex fractures, joint issues like arthritis, pinched nerves or spinal cord narrowing (spinal stenosis) as bleeding and blood clots, or infection and tumors. A myelogram (where a contrast dye is injected into the spinal column before the procedure) can be done with the CT scan. This test looks at the spinal cord, nerve roots, and nearby tissues, to see if a vertebra is pinching a nerve.

4. Bone Scan

A Bone Scan is a test to determine if back pain originates in the vertebrae of your spine. These tests can reveal bony lesions, metastases, or osteomyelitis (infection of the bone) and distinguish between dangerous and benign abnormalities in the spine.

All of these tests can certainly reveal physical damage from underuse, misuse, overuse, repeated injury, and repetitive trauma. They are most useful to rule out possible causes and narrow the scope of probable cause. If a diagnosis is accurate, it could determine root cause and indicate the most appropriate course of treatment. When the chosen treatment matches the original cause, healing can and will result.

For example, I once had a client, Jane, who came to me with knee pain after falling hard on both knees. After several weeks of therapeutic yoga, her pain got worse and not better, so I suggested she get an x-ray. It was a good thing she did, because the x-ray showed tiny bone chips around both kneecaps. The alignment exercises I taught her further lacerated the soft tissues. In fact, every time she walked, she caused more damage. In this case, surgically removing the bone chips was the best treatment for her. And after the surgery, the same exercises I previously taught her helped to strengthen her muscles and expedite a full recovery.

Remember, while a diagnosis can save time and money by providing a picture of what is happening inside the body, tests are not always conclusive, nor 100% accurate. False positives—scans suggesting the presence of a problem when none exists—can occur. Tests and results are a snapshot of a moment in time, while your body is made of living tissue that is in constant flux, improving or worsening every day. Also, x-rays and MRIs do not diagnose mental and emotional pain that can add significant stress to any injury, thus increasing one's pain levels.

Now what about those instances when a test is inconclusive, reveals nothing, and you find yourself back where you started? At least you have ruled out the big issues. Some doctors, upon finding no physical damage or abnormality in the spine, will insist back pain is caused by aging and will tell their patient there is nothing they can do to avoid or improve the situation.

While I'd agree that "aging" with poor posture over many decades can cause pain and problems, I completely disagree with the notion that one's health cannot be improved. If your test results are inconclusive, you'll definitely need to get more involved by learning what you can do to help yourself.

Curiously, between 80-90% of my clients never sought or received a diagnosis. When they do, I use the test results to refine and customize their BackCare Blueprint program. Yet, even without a diagnosis I am able to help my clients get out of pain 90% of the time. How do I do that? I use my own diagnostic skills. I listen to my clients describe their pain. I keenly observe how they move, breathe, speak, emote, and act. I look for the patterns most out of sync with the human blueprint and teach my clients how to return to balance. What I've noticed, regardless of whether or not a diagnosis exists, is when I apply sound alignment principles, my clients improve from a wide variety of structural issues. Their chronic pain resolves. Honestly, I teach everyone pretty much the same skills, and that's when I realized I could help more people with a book and video course. Why does this work? Because the original human design or blueprint is the same for everyone, and therefore, the same biomechanical principles of alignment and movement work for everyone to restore harmony and health. My job is pretty simple. I teach people the exact steps to put their body into a state of balance where it can and does heal itself. Since 75% of back pain is caused by structural misalignment (typically due to inactivity and poor postural habits), optimizing structural alignment is always a great place to begin. And in Part Three, I'll teach these steps to you!

PART ONE CONCLUSION

By now you understand the general conditions that can cause chronic back pain, have identified the main elements missing from your current approach, and see the value of a good medical diagnosis. You can see how a lack of patient knowledge, education, and participation thwart the healing process, how the lack of patient support and accountability to maintain new habits is crucial, and how a good diagnosis can point you towards the most appropriate path of healing. You've also learned that 75% of all back pain originates from structural misalignment, so learning to realign your body is a great place to start, regardless of if you have a diagnosis. Now let's dive deeper. What else will you need to shift in order to end the cycle of chronic back pain? As we transition into Part Two, we are going to examine how attitude, mindset and beliefs can make a big course correction in your healing journey.

PART TWO

COURSE CORRECTION
REORIENT YOUR APPROACH

Here in Part Two, you'll discover concepts to use as a guide to identify and shift your mindset and reorient your approach to back pain. By clearly seeing which attitudes are outdated, you can jumpstart the healing process from the inside out—the most effective way to guarantee long lasting results. In this section, I'll ask you to identify your main pattern of misalignment. When you see your postural misalignment clearly, the practices in Part Three will make more sense. Over time, you will gain the confidence to make small adjustments in mindset, posture, and breath to continually realign your body and reduce the pain.

CHAPTER 5

DITCH OLD PARADIGMS, ADOPT NEW ATTITUDES

"The definition of insanity is doing the same thing over and over and expecting different results." — *Albert Einstein*

In Part One, I mentioned that in order to alleviate your own suffering you'll need to make some changes. So, let us examine exactly what types of changes you can make. Even before you learn to realign your physical posture, it's crucial to adopt a new "inner stance." And before you change your attitude, it's vital to compare three healthcare models and recognize which one is your current default. Most people are stuck in the first paradigm. The work I do with clients moves them into the second model, but ultimately, it's up to them, and you, to step into the third.

1. DONE-FOR-YOU (DFY): FOREVER MANAGED HEALTH CARE

The existing 'status quo' medical model is the paradigm most people grew up with and rely upon today. It's what I call "Done-For-You" health care. When you're in pain, you visit your doctor, receive treatment and expect a cure. You don't have to do anything, change anything, or participate in any way, except to submit to "old guard" authority and standard treatments. As you may already know, this paradigm embeds the belief that doctors heal you and reinforces the idea that you cannot heal yourself. Allopathic medicine is limited for people with chronic conditions because it primarily masks or manages symptoms without addressing the root cause. This approach rarely cures chronic ailments.

2. DONE WITH YOU (DWY): INSPIRED SELF-CARE

If you are fortunate to have a health care practitioner who can recommend at-home practices or refers you to alternative therapists who do, you're better off than most people. In a Done-With-You model, you receive diagnosis and treatment as well as education about how to better care for yourself. Common advice typically includes standard recommendations for weight loss, physical therapy rehab, and exercise. While these suggestions are sound, they do not necessarily account for an individual's particular habits and specific needs, nor do they inspire change or create accountability for enacting positive change. Reading this book and following the practices herein, working privately with a knowledgeable practitioner who can guide you out of pain, or taking a course to learn at-home practices to reduce back pain yourself, are all examples of a "Done-With-You" approach.

Using this model, appropriate treatment combined with education and practice can inspire you to actively participate in your own healing. This will make your back feel better, and when it does, you'll have evidence that you can heal.

3. DO IT YOURSELF (DIY): EMPOWERED & FREE

Do-It-Yourself health care is where you finally become sovereign unto yourself. You've been inspired to take responsibility for your own health, to get educated and to take matters into your own hands. You've learned why you need to make specific changes, what changes you need to make and how to make them. You've stopped expecting someone else to fix you because you know how to help yourself. Now, you understand which old habits exacerbate pain, and which new habits relieve pain. This knowledge empowers and motivates you to consistently practice healthy alignment. Finally, you've learned to break the cycle of chronic back pain, but more importantly, you've learned how to get yourself out of pain. Congratulations!

Shifting from the old "DFY" paradigm to the "DWY" model and then to the "DIY" model takes time. It's common to fluctuate between these three paradigms as you learn healthy self-care routines for your spine. Sometimes you simply need extra help. The information in this book and in the accompanying video program will help you shift from the first to the second approach and become a more active and educated participant. Within this healing process, several important shifts in attitude are needed. Let's look at them now.

ADOPTING NEW ATTITUDES

During the crisis phase of my healing journey, the pain was constant and excruciating. I felt trapped in a maze with no way out! No matter which way I turned, I came face to face with pain that radiated from my lower back, across my buttocks, and down the back of my right leg. Over time, while in constant pain, I started to hate my own body. Constant pain sucked the joy out of my life, pain plummeted me down into a blackhole of emotion. One day my acupuncturist called out my poor attitude. "You need to stop thinking about your right leg as your 'bad' leg," he told me. Immediately, the light went on and I knew he was right. I realized how I contributed to pain by turning hate onto myself. It was an eye-opening moment for me, one that helped me make a huge course correction.

Still, I had an advantage: *I believed I could heal without pills, shots, or surgery.* But the majority of the 7+ million people with chronic back pain do not hold that belief. They haven't found the conviction or evidence that they can heal. If there's one shift to make right now, it is to open yourself up to the possibility, no matter how small, that "yes, I can heal myself."

What shifts in attitude might you need to make in order to find a viable exit strategy out of chronic back pain?

Write down your current beliefs about back pain here:

_____

_____

_____

SELF-TALK

"

I believed I could heal without pills, shots, or surgery.

Everyone I know—myself included—thinks, talks and refers to pain or illness in the first person. "I have always had this problem. My arthritis is flaring up. My cancer is incurable. My back pain is worse today. My bad back prevents me from driving, hiking, dancing, etc." Linguistically, we all use phrases I, me, my, and mine to describe our inner experience. But when we habitually fixate on pain in this way, we reinforce it as our primary identity. We embed pain into our psyche and cells. We claim it as our daily experience and when we do, we close the door to the possibility of regaining health. The crucial word here is "MY." When we view, speak, and identify with pain as "my" pain, we make things worse! If we're totally honest, we might see how pain has become a prized possession, one that's impossible to leave behind because we've formed an entire identity and negative narrative around it. I know I did!

Once I recognized how often I disrespected myself and shamed my body with harmful thoughts (my "bad" leg), I noticed how completely identified with pain I had become. I couldn't imagine who I'd be without pain because I kept calling it my own—MY pain. So, I adopted a radical strategy: I completely dropped my identity of pain and created a new language around it.

And now I suggest you do the same. Notice what words you use to describe back pain.

Write them down here:

_____

_____

_____

> **When we view, speak, and identify with pain as "my" pain, we make things worse!**

STOP IDENTIFYING "AS" PAIN. STOP CALLING PAIN "MY" PAIN.

Turn around and walk away from this mental habit and redefine a new relationship to your body and the internal sensations you experience day by day. I did, and you can, too.

My biggest turning point occurred during this monumental shift. The moment I stopped identifying with pain and using first person language (I, me, my, mine) was the moment I stepped onto the path of healing. I completely changed my negative mantra from "my" pain to "the" pain and then to "an experience of" pain.

I made a new habit of choosing different words: "Pain is present. I have an experience of pain. I notice a strong sensation in the back." Referring to pain objectively instead of in the first person. No more: "I, I, I, me, me, me, my, my, my, mine, mine, mine."

Try this step for the next week:

Be objective. Create space and stop referring to pain in the first person. Reframe your relationship to pain with neutral words like "an," "the," and "that." Stop saying "pain" and use words like "experience" "feeling" or "sensation." Become an objective witness of your body and what is occurring in each moment.

Instead of saying "My back is in pain. I am in pain," say, "There is an uncomfortable experience at this moment. I notice a strong sensation in the back. Something aggravates the lower back." This objectivity can interrupt your chronic identity and attachment to pain. Objectivity allows you to step back and perceive yourself through a bigger lens. It creates room to become curious about the nature and sensation of pain. It gives you the opportunity to ask: "Where does this pain come from? What part of my system is experiencing a sensation of pain? Is there actually a strong sensation now, or am I bracing against an experience that has not occurred?" Statements that put distance between you and "your" pain open up the space to explore the root causes of pain. And in this space, you'll be able to apply the pain-free practices in Part Three and shift your circumstance for the better.

OPTIMISM

Another strategy is to shift your self-talk from pessimism to optimism. You weren't always in pain, so tell yourself that you won't always experience pain. Affirm the other parts of your body that are healthy and fully functioning.

Every day say out loud: "My health IS improving. My back feels better. I AM getting stronger. I AM healing." This is so much healthier than thinking, "I'll never get well. I'm getting worse. My pain will never go away. I'm going to end up cripple." Science has proven how negative thoughts will make pain worse, and positive thoughts will relieve pain, so try to curb any mental negativity, as best you can and as soon as you notice it.

Positive affirmations can positively affect and speed the healing process. I bet you've already blamed yourself for being stuck in this situation (I know I did), so why not try a different tack? Give yourself a huge boon by instilling a message of hope and positivity as your new mindset. Give yourself a high-five for reading this book, assuming a new attitude, and stepping on the road to wellness.

Write down your three most negative beliefs about back pain.

1. I am _____.

2. I am _____.

3. I am _____.

Now rewrite each one as a positive affirmation.

1. I am _____.

2. I am _____.

3. I am _____.

> **"**
>
> *Every day say out loud: "My health IS improving. My back feels better. I AM getting stronger. I AM healing."*

We've discussed several positive approaches you can adopt today to turn your life around. The importance of shifting from constant reliance on a "Done-For-You" approach of medicine to embark upon a "Do-It-Yourself" path of empowerment. The necessity to alter negative self-talk into an optimistic attitude and the benefit of reframing pain as an observer. These inner changes will help you to break the cycle of chronic back pain.

Now, let's reimagine the chronic pain model as a new model of wellness.

You are at the heart of this healthy paradigm! Your desire to live pain-free and your willingness to take responsibility for your own health are key. Becoming an active participant in your healing journey is crucial. This new model outlines the basic pathway to freedom from back pain. And although creating proper alignment is primary to healing pain caused by structural misalignment, you really can start with any area, because they are all interconnected. Shifting one area creates an opening that can and will shift all others.

Adopting a positive mental outlook first goes a long way. The idea that you can heal yourself is completely new to some people. The stronger your belief in this truth, the happier you will feel and the faster you will heal.

Happiness will keep you motivated to practice the alignment and breath practices in Part Three. And as you become savvy with them, your habits will become healthier, you'll make better choices — all of which will help patterns of chronic pain to dissolve.

Once you're familiar and comfortable with the concepts and practices of the BackCare Blueprint program, you'll notice that certain areas may need more of your attention than others. Once you're established in the wellness model, you can choose the practice that supports you best, and as you do, your health will keep spiraling upwards.

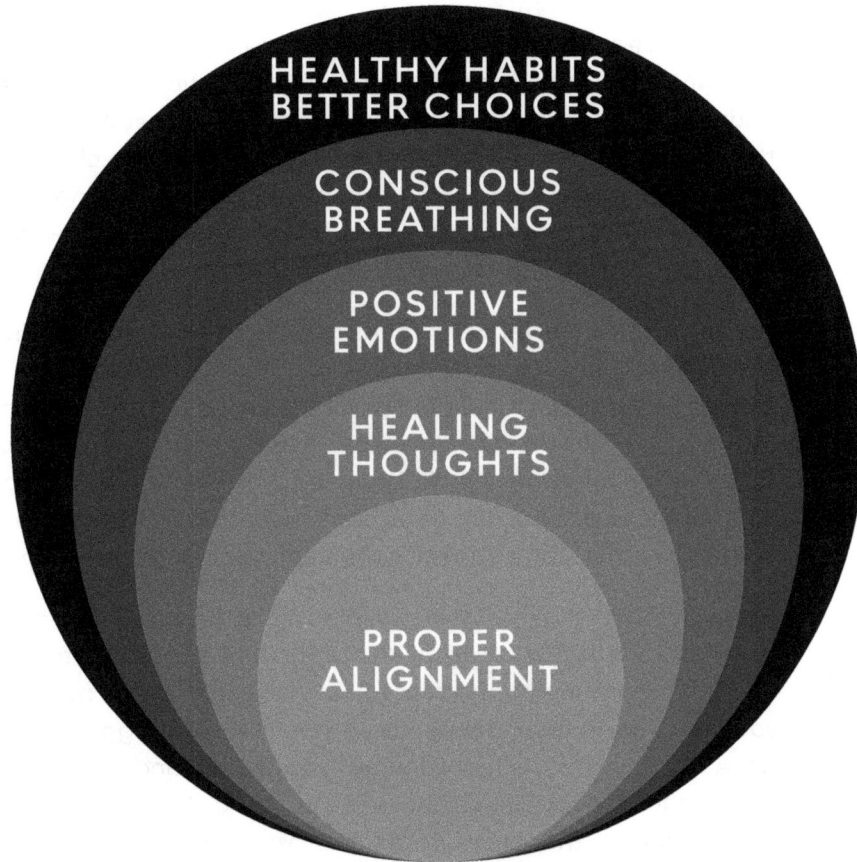

HEALTHY HABITS
BETTER CHOICES

CONSCIOUS
BREATHING

POSITIVE
EMOTIONS

HEALING
THOUGHTS

PROPER
ALIGNMENT

WELLNESS MODEL

It's also wise to embrace change and set realistic goals. You haven't had back pain your whole life, so you needn't suffer with it for the remainder of your life. If you've endured pain for many years, you might expect that it will take time to acquire the new habits that will help you heal. In working with clients I've noticed that it generally takes between 8–12 weeks of consistent and mindful practice to change old patterns and establish new ones. In three months, you can learn to get yourself out of pain! Isn't that great news?

Embracing change by welcoming new habits and supplanting old habits with positivity will enhance your healing experience. My personal mantra for embracing change is, "small shifts yield big results." Like the tortoise in the child's story, a slow steady effort wins the race. If you can make one small change today and maintain that change tomorrow, you'll be able to make another change next week, and another the week after. But if you don't make that first step, it will take a miracle for you to heal. Thus, commitment, consistency, and dedication are required.

There's another essential component to make the transition from a "Done-For-You" paradigm to the "Done-With-You" approach and finally to the "Do-It-Yourself" model. It's extremely important to have an experienced guide who's stood where you stand, one who understands what it's like to struggle in constant pain as you do. A healer who's made the journey successfully and knows the terrain with all its pitfalls and setbacks like the back of their hand. A mentor who knows what it takes to descend into the valley of despair, cross a river of pain, and climb the mountain back to radiant health. Without the right quality of support, you could be stuck in a cycle of chronic back pain, forever. Finally, I wholeheartedly recommend you view this entire process as an adventurous journey; returning to a place of health you haven't been in a long time. A place that is still familiar enough to see, feel, touch or imagine. In Chapter 9, I'll guide you through a visualization to help you get clear on what a pain-free life could look and feel like for you.

A RECIPE FOR SUCCESS

The recipe for success is simple: get educated, get support,
and get started!

To make a successful trek, you need new strategies.
Ones that lead you back to wholeness.

To effectively heal chronic back pain, it's important to:

1. Stop expecting others to fix your back.

2. Believe that you can heal chronic back pain.

3. Exclaim out loud: "I am getting better every day."

4. Stop identifying with "my" pain, instead refer to "that" sensation.

5. Embrace the process of change as a personal healing journey.

6. Take small steps, one at a time, and get support when you need it.

7. When you finish reading this book, put these practices to good use.

Next, let's look at your physical posture and discover why it might be
the source of back pain.

CHAPTER 6

THE COCKTAIL POSE — IDENTIFY YOUR PAINFUL POSTURE

"Every moment of our life can be the beginning of great things." — *Joseph Pilates*

In this chapter, you'll identify one posture that most closely matches your habitual stance. This priceless knowledge will help you see yourself more clearly and enable you to apply the practices in Part Three with more precision. Although your posture is unique to you, there are several main archetypes of poor posture common to the human collective. As you view the pictures below and read their descriptions, try to ascertain your primary misalignment. I have coined a term for the way people habitually stand as their "cocktail pose." When you're hanging out with friends or standing in line, how do you typically stand or slouch? What is the shape of your spine? When you sit down, do you have the same pattern or a different one?

To begin, let's look at an ideal posture—the natural blueprint of the human body that keeps you out of pain and feeling healthy and happy. Then, let's look at the most common postural misalignments, so you can identify yours.

The Pain-Free Posture (Ideal):

In an ideal, pain-free posture, your neck and lower back have a natural inward curve while your thoracic spine and sacrum have a natural outward curve. In this position, notice how the ears, shoulders, hip sockets, knee joints and ankles form a straight vertical line. This plumb line allows gravity to ground effectively into the earth instead of getting jammed up in the spinal vertebrae and stressing the joints. In an optimal posture, the spine not only acts as a grounding rod for gravity, but it also becomes a conduit of vital energy, promoting balanced energy flow through your entire physical body. An optimal posture allows you to return to optimal health and generates feelings of confidence, ease, poise, and inner strength at the same time. But when gravity gets the better of you and your spine collapses, all four curves are negatively affected and the risk for back pain increases. In Part Three, I'll teach you how to create your own pain-free posture.

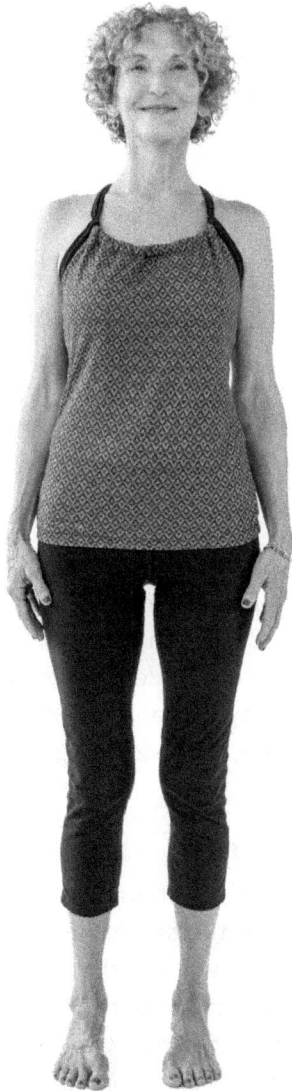

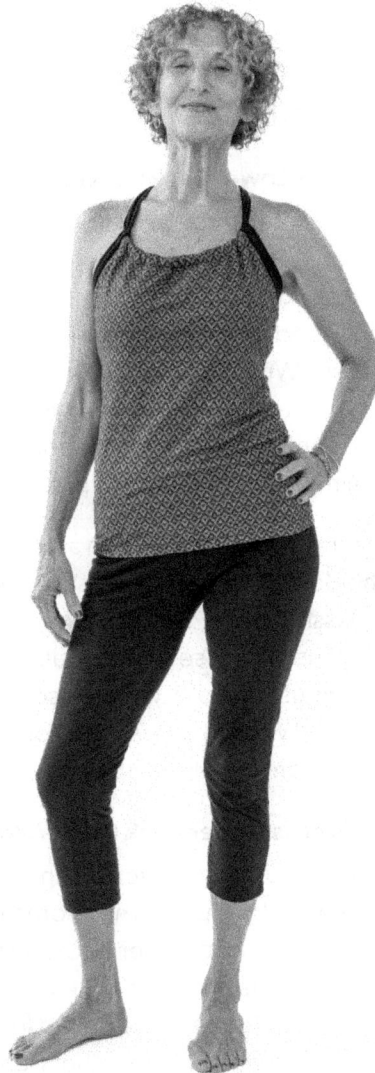

Pain-Free Pose

Cocktail Pose

"

The spine not only acts as a grounding rod for gravity, but it also becomes a conduit of vital energy, promoting balanced energy flow.

THE SIX PAINFUL POSTURES:

1. Lumbar Lordosis (Excess Lower Back Curve)

Lumbar Lordosis is a fancy term for overarching your lower back. It's an excessive curve where the lumbar vertebrae shift forward from the central axis. The position a gymnast takes when sticking the perfect landing—butt pushed back, deep curve in the lower back, belly and chest pushed proudly forward—is a good example of extreme lumbar lordosis. While it's the perfect end to a competitive floor routine, it's a terrible position to embody throughout your life. It puts excess strain into the lower back and will definitely make your whole back hurt because you're over-contracting the spinal muscles and putting pressure on the nerves.

After attending one of my yoga classes, Nan asked for help outside of class because she had issues with her lower back. In the first session, I identified the main postural misalignment—the classic hollow back (lumbar lordosis) posture—that put strain into her lower back. In just a few sessions, I taught Nan how to reduce the excess curve in her lower back using both yoga poses and everyday movements. After finding such a simple "fix" which I share with you in Part Three, Nan was delighted that her lower back pain completely disappeared.

2. Thoracic Kyphosis (Excess Upper Back Curve/Slouchy Shoulders)

Thoracic Kyphosis is a term used to describe an excess curve of the thoracic spine. While kyphosis is the natural shape of the thoracic spine (and the same shape as the sacrum), when the middle and upper back muscles become weak or the bones decay due to osteoporosis, the spine slouches, and the natural curve of the upper back becomes exaggerated. As the spine collapses, the front of the chest (sternum) caves in, the middle of the spine pushes further behind the central axis than normal, the shoulders round down, and the chin droops towards the chest. A dowager's hump would be a good example of an excessive thoracic curve. In addition to

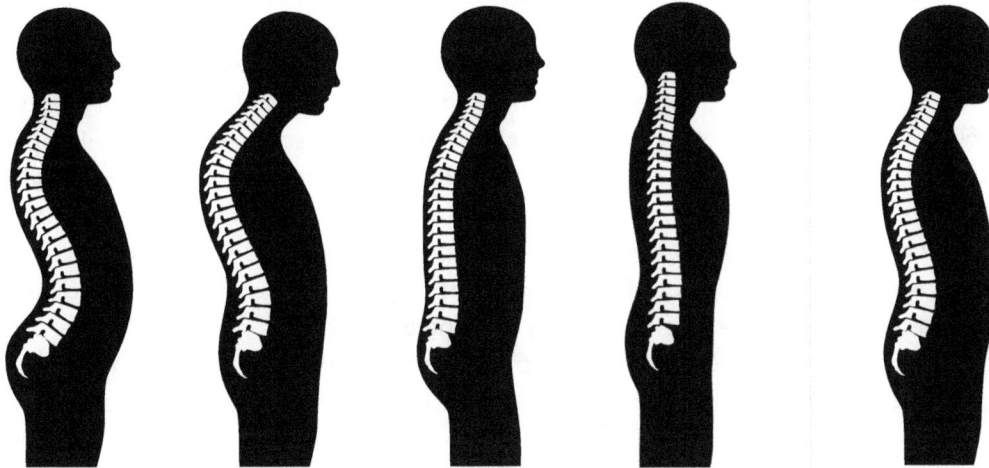

1. Lordosis   *2. Kyphosis*   *3. Flat Back*   *4. Military*   *Healthy*

exacerbating mid-back and neck pain, breathing deeply is also impaired while in this position, and the lack of lung-filling oxygen can make you feel unhappy, sad, or even depressed.

3. Flat Back (Reverse Lumbar Curve)

A flat back or reverse curve typically refers to the lower back, and only rarely applies to the upper back. In this position, the curve of the lumbar spine is diminished, flattened, or reversed putting excess pressure on the vertebrae, discs, and nerve endings that run from the lower back down into the sacrum. When standing in this position, there is a tendency to push the pelvis and tailbone forward, and in the process, tightening the hips and flattening the curve of the lower back. The knees lock to compensate and maintain balance. This is a very common position among young women, putting extra gravitational weight and stress into the sacral-iliac (SI) joints—a primary structural cause of sacral pain. Most people who sit for prolonged periods do so with severely misaligned posture. It's common for those who have "weak butt" syndrome or "sitter's disease" to have a flat back or reversed curve because they slouch the pelvis backwards and sit on the sacrum instead of the sitting bones. If you love to end your day relaxing on the couch, it's likely that you too are reversing the curve of your lumbar spine. Chronically flattening one's lower back can lead to lower back pain now, and herniated discs or degenerative disc disease later on in life.

4. Military Posture (Excess Extension/Flat Upper Back)

When using military posture, every muscle in the body is tight and the spine is rigid, overly pushing the chest forward and throwing the shoulders back. The chin is also pushed forward, straining the neck. In this 'ready for action' position, the excess tension in the back muscles restricts the breath and hardens the body. Standing at attention has its place in the military, but not in a civilian's everyday life.

My client, Rani, came to me complaining about lower back pain whenever she sat, hiked, or snowshoed. Thinking the military position was the correct way to stand, Rani was shocked when her massage therapist told her that constantly over-contracting the back muscles whenever she "stood up straight and sucked in her stomach," were causing her issues. So, I taught her to reverse her tendency to overuse the lower back muscles and underuse the abdominal muscles. Once we sorted that out, Rani understood how to properly adjust her posture and enjoy the outdoors without strain or pain.

5. Scoliosis (C and S Curves)

Here, the curves of the spine move out of alignment on the sagittal plane which divides the body in half from left to right. Scoliosis differs from kyphosis and lordosis because in both of those conditions, the spine moves forward and back along the frontal plane. Typically, scoliosis is caused by misalignment in the lower body or imbalance in the pelvis and weakness in the muscles of the spine. Scoliosis can occur in the neck, middle back, or lower back. Sometimes scoliosis is a congenital issue, often an issue of underuse.

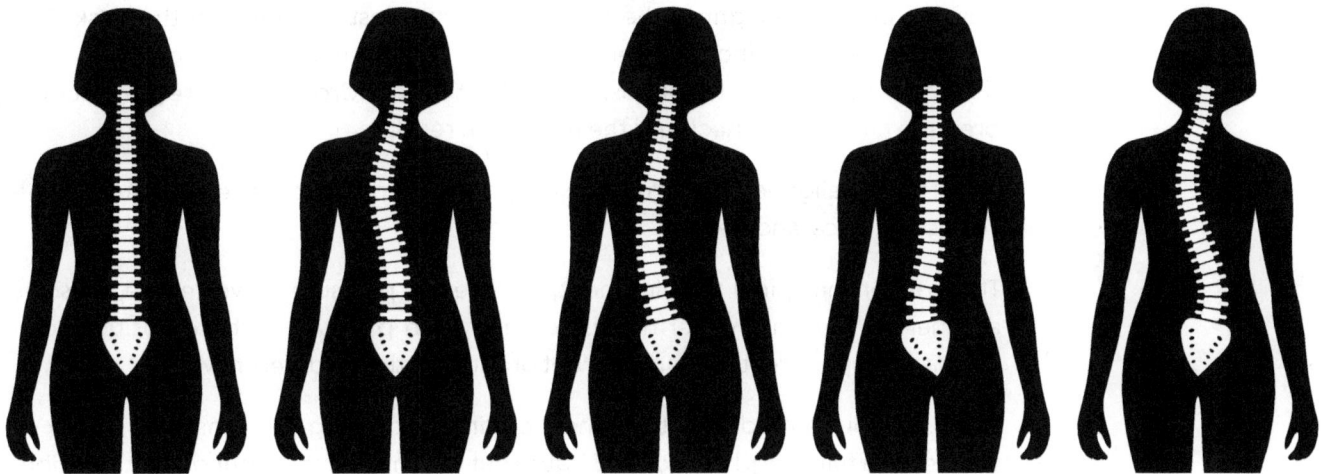

Healthy Spine   *C-shaped Curves*   *S-shaped Curve*

In a "C" shaped curve, the spine bends in one direction (arcing to the right or left) and can even overlap two areas of the spine (the cervical and thoracic or thoracic and lumbar vertebrae). An "S" curve is made up of two "C" shaped curves that move in opposite directions. One part of the spine bends to the right and the other bends to the left. So, you could have a right leaning thoracic and left leaning lumbar, or left leaning thoracic and a right leaning lumbar. The same is true for the neck and upper back.

6. Text Neck

With a text neck (tech neck), the posture and spinal curves are typically well-positioned, but the head drops forward and the chin tucks down to the chest. This position puts the weight of the skull into the smallest vertebrae of the neck. This distortion can also pinch the cervical nerves, causing numbness or radiating pain down the arms and into the hands. The further the head drops, the more gravitational pressure falls into the neck and the more pain results.

ALL of the misaligned positions in the image that follows put uneven pressure on the vertebrae, discs, and nerves.

The greater the spinal misalignment, the greater pressure on vertebrae, muscles and nerves, and the higher the risk of injury and pain. All of these positions can diminish proper breathing and disrupt organ function in different ways.

Now that you've read about the most common standing patterns, take a look at yourself in a full-length mirror and figure out which pattern is your default position. You may have a combination of more than one pattern.

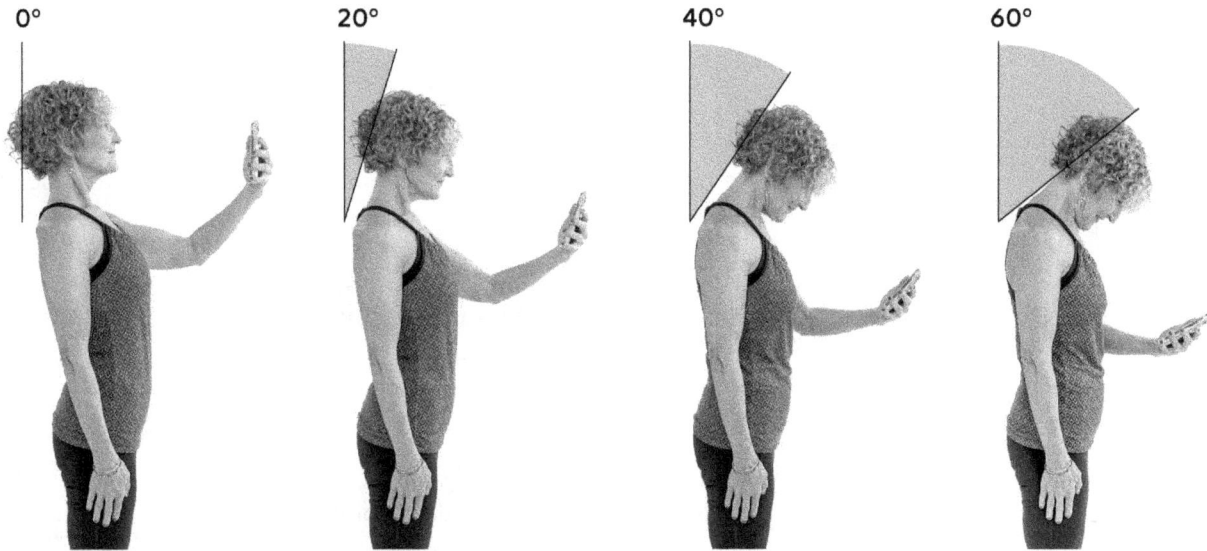

0°   20°   40°   60°

Text Neck

Write YOUR "Cocktail Pose" down here:

_____

_____

Now check to see if you have the same pattern when sitting down.

If you have a different pattern, write it here:

_____

_____

Can you see why a particular part of your back hurts because of the way you stand or sit?

That's really important information to know. Once you recognize your pattern, it is easier to reshape your posture and bring your spinal curves back into balance. Now, let's reshape the way you think about pain!

PAIN AS A MESSENGER

Pain is a love message from your body that points to imbalance. Pain is a great teacher, when observed closely, can lead you from suffering to wholeness.

What would you discover if you listened to the intrinsic wisdom stored in your spine and held within the sensation of pain? We all agree that pain is personal and subjective, and also something we'd all rather avoid than experience. While most people focus on getting rid of pain, my approach is radically different. I prefer to study pain and learn from it. In my experience, the way out of chronic pain is to step into it—using pain to get to know yourself, your patterns, your habits, your triggers. Using this information, you can then create new habits, so the message from pain works for you and not against you. By getting to know what the pain is telling you, you'll be able to get yourself out of pain. And when you do, you'll start to enjoy life again.

Pain as Best Friend, Not Worst Enemy

What if you were to personify pain? What would he or she look like? What would Pain be telling you? Would it be trying to hurt or help you? One thing I learned as I worked my way out of chronic sciatica and lower back pain was this: pain is my friend. An ally. When I made pain my partner on the road to recovery, it became my Best Friend, Forever. Pain told me when I was "in" or "out" of alignment. It rewarded

> " ——
>
> *Pain is a love message from your body that points to imbalance. Pain is a great teacher, when observed closely, can lead you from suffering to wholeness.*

72

me when I was doing something right (less pain), and nudged me when I was doing something wrong (more pain). Pain scolded me whenever I sat too long or slouched my spine. Most of all, pain never lied to me! Pain always sent me a clear, straightforward message to adjust my posture, engage my muscles, get up and walk around, or do a few therapeutic stretches.

All of these strategies reconnected my brain and body and restored healthy cellular pulsation, flow and function, and returned a normal rhythm to the affected tissues— which ultimately eliminated both my sciatic and back pain. Truth be told, once you stop resisting pain, you can start dialoguing with it. As you dialogue with pain, you, too, will receive important information that helps you tap your inner wisdom and gain access to the healing powers of your body.

Eventually, misalignment can become a great ally. Your spine is already telling you to change your habits. Pain motivates you to discover both the root cause and the remedy. So, let's get a sense of what pain is already telling you!

LANGUAGE OF THE BODY

In this section, I'd like to give you a feeling for the language of the body and how it communicates. Pain is subjective and so its voice is distinct to you. If you are sensitive, a particular sensation may bother you a lot, but might not bother someone else at all. When you willingly receive the messages that your body communicates through pain (instead of automatically ignoring them or dulling them by popping a painkiller), you'll gather useful information about what is out of balance and you'll be better able to choose appropriate practices (from Part Three) to restore balance.

Let's imagine that every sensation or pain occurring in a specific part of your body or within a certain type of tissue has a unique voice. That voice draws your mind

66 ——————

Once you stop resisting pain, you can start dialoguing with it.

73

towards itself—the part most in need of attention. A tiny whisper might indicate a small issue that you could tend to now or later. An insistent voice warns you of a pressing issue, which, if left unattended, could grow worse. A screaming bloody murder voice clearly indicates the presence of a severe issue or trauma requiring immediate attention and medical care.

Let's start with the tiny voice and examine the progression of pain from mild to intense. These first three sensations have a lot in common, varying by degree and subjectivity.

Stiffness

Spinal stiffness is typically the first indication that something is out of balance. Waking up stiff in the morning is very common. During sleep, while your body lays still, lacking movement and circulation, the tissues dehydrate. Dehydration can contribute to morning stiffness. And a common habit with so many people is to wake up stiff, drink coffee, drive to work, sit for 8–10 hours, and then return home and rest on the couch. Repeating these habits of a sedentary lifestyle day after day instills a pattern of stiffness in your body. Over time stiffness—repeated and reoccurring—becomes embedded as a chronic pattern. In addition, the habitual way you sit at work stresses your lower back, upper back and/or neck, so even an inconsequential misalignment in your spine could eventually become locked into a chronic pattern. Although we think morning stiffness is normal, this tiny voice is actually your body's early warning sign that both underuse and misuse exist. It issues you a clear message: "Get up and move around before stiffness gets worse."

Tightness/Constriction/Tension

When stiffness progresses, the sensation feels more akin to tightness or constriction. When experiencing tightness or tension, a group of muscles (rather than a single muscle) gets weaker and the surrounding fascia (connective tissue) which wraps around and through the muscles, organs, tissues becomes more constricted, limiting the range of motion in a larger area. Stiffness spreads from a localized spot to a wider area and the sensation becomes more noticeable and more bothersome. Perhaps you wiggle your spine to loosen up your back in response. The ideal response here—for both your muscles and fascia—is movement and stretching, not popping a pill! It's worth noting that what we commonly call "tight" muscles are more often weak rather than overly-developed. Weak muscles shorten and create trigger points or knots in the fiber. So, this louder voice also indicates underuse and misuse and the need to take action: "We're more uncomfortable than before. We need more movement not less."

Dull, Achy, Sore

Tightness and tension that result from serious lack of exercise can cause muscles to atrophy. When this occurs, everyday chores like lifting and bending make the back muscles feel achy and sore. A frequent dull or heavy sensation in the muscles and fascia from sedentary lifestyle of underuse is also common. Lack of movement deprives the cells and muscles of oxygen, so your body calls out for attention. This louder more insistent voice comes as a sense of heaviness, dullness, or fatigue because not enough blood is pumped through the muscles and so stagnation, which follows stiffness and constriction, sets in. Movement is slow and cumbersome. Dullness, heaviness, achiness and soreness indicate underuse or misuse, so again the message is to get up and move around. Sometimes soreness is an issue of overuse, where you've exhausted the muscles and they just need some good rest.

Sudden/Sharp/Piercing/Stabbing/Throbbing

A sudden sharp pain message typically arises at the moment of impact or injury. You move too quickly and pull a muscle or lift something too heavy and tear a tendon or ligament. Or you fall down and bruise a bone. Throbbing could also indicate a bone fracture. Now you're really in a lot of pain! This voice cries out loudly for immediate attention. The more serious the injury, the more intense the pain, the louder the voice. Throbbing or irritating pain could also arise from inflammation or osteoarthritis in the facet joints of the back of the spine. So, this voice could indicate issues with the muscles, tendons, ligaments, joints or bones . . . but not with the nerves. "We (tissues) are hurt and need some extra care right now."

Burning/Numbness/Tingling/Radiating/Prickly

A burning, numbing, tingling sensation sends an irrefutable message that the nerves are inflamed or injured. Nerve pain can be excruciating and often radiates outward away from the point of injury. It can stop you in your tracks and make you cry. A bulging or ruptured disk puts pressure on the nerves, while inflammation, a slipped vertebrae or misalignment can pinch a nerve. A misalignment of the lumbar vertebrae can trigger the sciatic nerve, radiating a burning sensation down the lower back, buttocks, backs of the thighs, into the shins and feet. Any sensation that feels like your body is on fire is a signal from the nerves. These messages are not to be overlooked nor taken lightly. This voice screams, "Something is really wrong here. We need immediate help. We need soothing."

What's important to know about nerves is that the area of pain may not be the same location as the problem. Take a look at the dermatome chart and you'll see the areas of pain that are triggered from misalignment or damage to specific vertebrae or areas of the body.

NOTE: Sudden, Acute Weakness/Buckling/ Numbness of the Legs

If you experience sensations of weakness, buckling, or numbness in the legs combined with severe lower back pain, sciatica in one or both legs, and loss of bladder or bowel control, within a 24-hour period, seek emergency medical care immediately! You may have a serious condition called cauda equina, which impacts the nerve roots of the lumbar and sacrum area and can lead to paralysis if left untreated.

...

Now that you've identified the type of sensation you're feeling, it's important to locate the origin of the sensation using the dermatome chart that follows. And to help you further decipher the language of your body, I've created a questionnaire. The act of contemplating these questions will deepen the connection to your own body and receive valuable information-instead of ignoring the issue or masking it with painkillers.

Dermatome chart

The dermatome chart is a very useful tool which can help you identify a specific vertebra or vertebrae causing pain in another part of your body. By using this chart, you can see how neck issues could be the source of pain in the arms, or an issue in the sacrum could radiate pain down the backs of the buttocks and legs. Start with the area of the pain and work back to see which vertebrae may be affected. Bear in mind, this does not necessarily give you the root cause (because there could be many issues within a particular vertebrae), but it does give you a big clue and indicates where to adjust your spine.

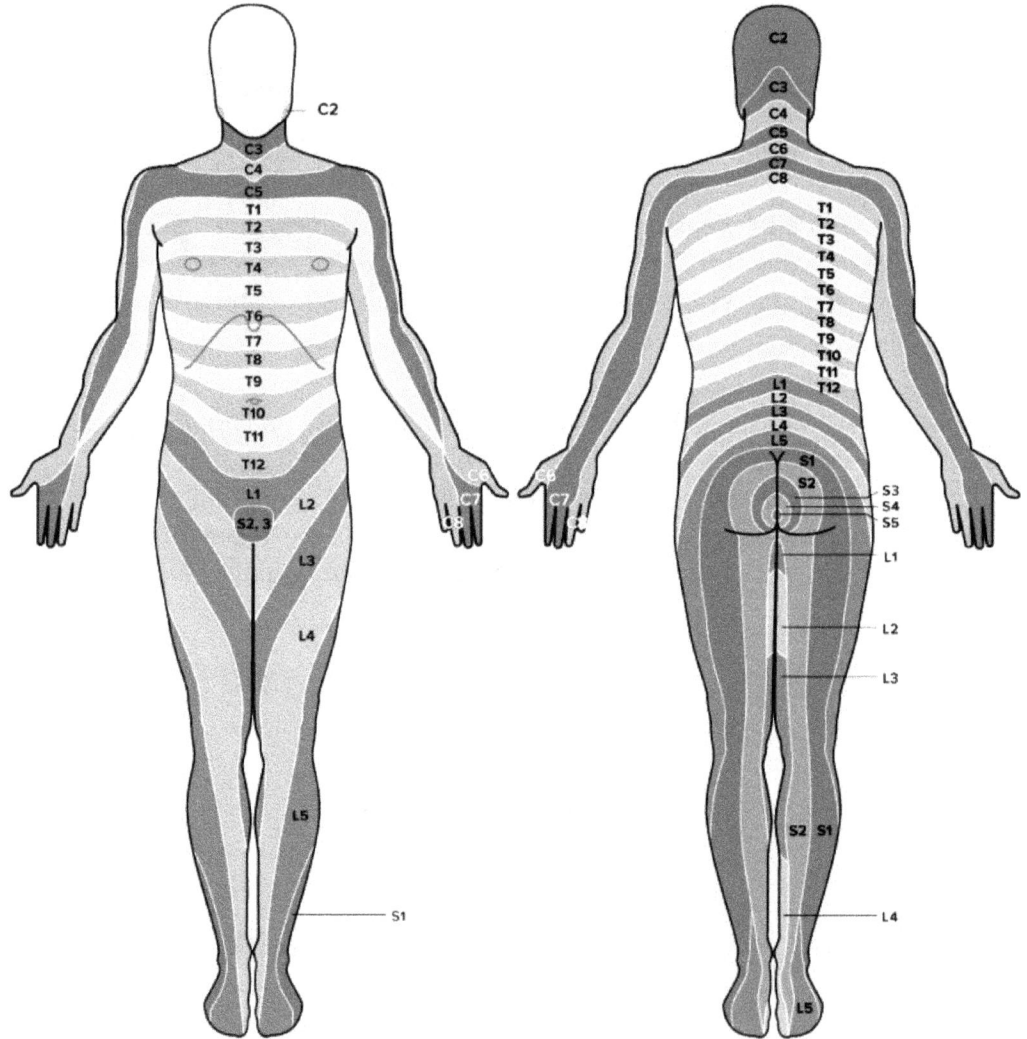

Anterior view

Posterior view

Consider these questions as you assess your situation.

Rate the current pain on a scale of 1–10? (low to high)

1. Severity: Is the sensation mild, moderate, or severe?

2. Location: Do you feel the sensation locally, in a specific spot that you can put your finger on, or do you feel the sensation in a general area? Is the pain changeable, moving around or is pain static, staying in the same place?

3. Which vertebra relates to the area of pain in the dermatome chart? (see previous page)

4. Depth: Is the sensation superficial (layer of skin), medium (layers of fat, muscle, nerve), or deep (layer of bone)?

5. Frequency/Duration: How often do you experience this sensation? Is your experience intermittent, constant, or variable? How long does pain typically last?

6. Description: How would you describe the sensation: stiff, tight/tense, dull/heavy/achy/sore, sharp/throbbing, intense/fiery/numb/tingly, or excruciating/unbearable/unrelenting?

7. Time of Day: What time of day does the sensation occur? When is it worse? Better? Gone?

8. Cause: What positions or movements make pain worse? Better?

9. Which positions reduce pain: moving, resting, standing, sitting, lying down, other?

10. Excess/Deficiency: Is pain caused by too much activity, strain, stress, or too little exercise, breath, positivity, or proper alignment?

11. Treatment: Is there any movement that reliably relieves this pain? If so, what?

Remember, you are learning to observe your body and communicate with pain, so not having an answer to some of these questions is perfectly okay.

Now, let's look at pain from another angle and try to determine what tissues might be chronically strained, injured, or traumatized.

SITES OF INJURY, TYPES OF PAIN:

The following list can help you think more deeply about the cause of your back pain, and what tissues might be affected by the type of pain you experience. This information is NOT meant to diagnose. It's only meant to provide examples of possible sources of back pain and get you thinking about your own situation.

Disc (Herniated/Bulging/Ruptured/Degenerated)

Spinal discs make space between adjoining vertebrae to prevent bone-on-bone rubbing, and act as shock absorbers to gravity during physical activity. When discs become compressed from poor posture or misalignment they can protrude or bulge. If they bulge forward, pain will be non-existent. But if they bulge backwards, you'll feel pain since the spinal nerves are located on the back of the vertebrae. Degenerated disc disease (DDD) is a common diagnosis. Sometimes it's used as a catch-all when the cause of back pain remains unknown. DDD can result from years of wear and tear, an issue of misuse, underuse, or overuse, or result from osteoporosis as the vertebrae deteriorate. When any of these happen, more pressure falls onto the discs.

Sensation: Burning or cold sensation, stinging, sharpness, numbness, weakness, or pain from your back down through your legs and feet are common symptoms of disc problems.

Nerve

When a misaligned posture or DDD compresses the nerves or if the nerves are damaged in an accident, the degree of pain will vary depending on the type of injury. But since nerve pain is unlike other pains, it is easily assessed.

Sensation: hot, intense, fiery, prickly, stinging, radiating, numbing, shooting, burning, searing, scorching, as if your nerves are on fire.

Muscle/Tendon

The spine uses many muscles to both move and stabilize the vertebrae. The deepest muscles look like shoelaces, crisscrossing the back from neck to the lower back. The next layer (paraspinals) run vertically up and down both sides of the spine. All muscles and the tendons that attach them to the bones can be too tight or too loose. They can be bruised or strained from overuse, sprained or torn from misuse, or achy, stiff and sore from underuse. Muscles that are bruised physically hurt when touched. Strained, sprained, or torn muscles tend to hurt the more you move and hurt less when you rest. Muscles that are weak and underused feel stronger with activity. Muscles that are too contracted from overuse feel better when stretched.

Sensation: Achy, sore, tender when bruised or strained. Sharp, jabbing, throbbing, intense when torn.

Fascia

Fascia is a type of connective tissue that wraps around and through the body like a web. Fascia is sticky and can become bound to other tissues restricting range and ease of movement. Tight fascia and tight muscles go hand in hand. They both feel better with movement and stretching.

Sensation: bound, tight, sore, heavy, thick, sticky.

Ligament

Ligaments connect bones to bones. They do not have a large blood supply, are very slow to heal and pain can linger for months. The ligaments of the spine run vertically along the spinal ridge.

Sensation: sore and achy when strained or bruised; constant deep, intense ache when sprained or torn.

Facet Joint

Muscles/tendons move bones, ligaments hold bones in position to protect the joints. The spinal facet joints can get stuck in a misaligned position from repeated poor posture or inflamed from osteoarthritis.

Sensation: sore, tight, stiff, immobile when misaligned. Throbbing, intense, hot, burning from arthritis.

Bone

If you've fractured a vertebra or rib, the sensation varies depending on the severity of the break. Broken bones hurt constantly with or without movement and hurt more when weight-bearing and movement occurs. Sensation: mild throb with hairline fracture; excruciating deep pain when a bone shears off, is broken in half, or crushed.

Cyst

Benign or malignant cysts on the vertebrae or back of the ribs can put pressure on the spinal nerves causing mild to intense pain.

Skin

The nerve endings in the skin of the back can become triggered, causing tingly or prickly sensation or numbness.

Organ

Dysfunction or disease in any of the internal organs could affect the way your spine feels. Organ sensation can vary depending on the organ, ranging from mild to intense, achy to sharp, hot or cold.

Bear in mind, one injured part could affect another, so mixed types of pain are pretty common with spinal injury or accident, but our focus continues to be on pain caused by structural misalignment. Now let's continue with our investigation of chronic back pain.

FOUR MOST COMMON BACK ISSUES

Degenerative Disc Disease (DDD)

Degenerative Disc Disease (DDD) happens when discs thin out, tear, herniate or rupture. With thinning or tearing, pain is localized. A herniated or ruptured disc may radiate pain out the arms if the cervical discs are affected. Pain radiating down the lower body is often caused by sciatica or piriformis syndrome. Pain levels may vary through the day. Relief will differ according to location and cause by bending forward, backward, spinal traction, walking or laying down.

Pinched Nerve

Pain from a pinched nerve is mostly felt in the legs but can be felt in the upper back or neck, or simultaneously in the legs, back and neck. Typically, this pain is worse in the legs than the upper back. Nerve pain is aggravated by sitting and bending forward and relieved by bending backwards, but in an acute stage could be worsened by back bending. If this is the case, pain can be reduced by lying on the belly or lying on the back with a pillow under the backs of the knees.

Facet Joint Pain

Facet Joint pain that is located in the lower back often spreads down into the buttocks and legs, just like disc pain. Pain located in the facet joints of the neck shoots across the shoulders and upper back, but not down the arms. This pain is also intermittent—on and off—throughout the day. You can tell the difference between disc pain and facet joint pain because the movements that aggravate the first, relieve the second. Facet joint pain is worse when bending backwards, standing, or walking for long periods of time and reduced by sitting down or bending forward.

Sacroiliac Joint Pain

Pain is located on the affected sacroiliac joint (right or left) and can feel dull, achy, or sharp. Pain can move into the buttocks, thighs, groin, or upper back. Imbalanced posture such as standing unevenly on two legs, standing on one leg, sitting with one leg crossed over the other, climbing stairs or moving from sitting to standing can trigger pain. It might feel worse in the morning and improve during the day. Symmetric movements can relieve this pain, as can creating balance in the pelvis and lower back.

ADDITIONAL BACK ISSUES

Scoliosis

Scoliosis is a curvature of the spine that is abnormal. A "C" curve is where the spine shifts laterally to the right or left side. An "S" curve shifts side-to-side both to the right and to the left. Curves that exaggerate the natural shape of a front to back curve are called Kyphotic when the thoracic spine is overly rounded, and lordotic when the lumbar curve is too deep. Pain can be relieved by lengthening the spine, traction, and strengthening specific muscles to decrease the curvature.

Osteoarthritis

Osteoarthritis is the most common form of arthritis, affecting the joints of the hands, knees, hips, and spine of millions of people worldwide. Also called "degenerative joint disease," osteoarthritis is an issue of wear-and-tear. The protective cartilage covering the ends of the bones breaks down over time, causing pain, stiffness, swelling and inflammation. The amount of pain you might feel likely increases over time as cartilage continues to degrade. The resulting sensation can shift from achy to sore and sore to intense, but is not fiery like nerve pain.

Arthritis can be relieved by creating space in the joints and applying gentle movement in all directions.

Spinal Stenosis

Spinal stenosis is a narrowing of the spinal canal and can be caused by several things, including osteoarthritis, DDD, herniated disc, thickened ligaments, and spinal deformity. A dull, heavy or achy pain is located in the center of the back and in the legs, although pain is typically worse in the legs. It occurs off and on with activity. Pain from spinal stenosis is always worse with movement and walking for more than a few minutes can trigger pain. Pain is often relieved by changing positions, sitting and bending forward.

Spondylolisthesis

Due to injury, accident, or shock of impact from strenuous exercise, a vertebra is pushed forward of the ones above and below. This pain is exacerbated by twisting, lifting, bending and almost any activity. Pain can be felt in the lower back, buttocks, legs, or both. Diffused weakness of the legs can be experienced when walking or standing for lengthy periods. Pain is relieved by lying on the back to stabilize the vertebrae and through non-weight-bearing exercises like swimming.

Ligamentum Flavum

The ligamentum flavum is a highly elastic ligament that runs the length of the spine from C2–S1. It sits inside the spinal canal between the spinal processes (bone) and the spinal cord. Here, it prevents excessive gaps or separation between the vertebrae. It also functions like a muscle, pulling the spine upright into vertical alignment from a forward bending position. Damage to this ligament can cause thickening or swelling (hypertrophy) which can put pressure on the spinal cord and into the nerves. It can also become overstretched and put pressure on the nerve roots and disc when extending the spine. Forward bends can relieve this type of back pain.

Bone Spurs

Bone spurs on the spine (or elsewhere) can form in response to the inflammation caused by osteoarthritis. When this occurs, chronic inflammation breaks down the cartilage that cushions the ends of bones. The body, as it attempts to repair loss of cartilage, creates bone spurs in the damaged area. Unweighting the joints can relieve some pain, as can dietary measures to reduce inflammation.

CONCLUSION

While there are many things that can go wrong with your spine, the ones listed above can be improved by correcting postural misalignment and changing the habits that trigger these issues.

Again, a diagnosis can provide valuable information; knowing what is wrong informs you on how to proceed. But in order to proceed, you need to see your habitual postural misalignment (cocktail pose) clearly, understand what message the pain is trying to tell you, and be willing to reframe pain from enemy to friend.

Over the next two chapters, we'll look at the anatomy of the spine and the breath and investigate the seven types of movement. This information will equip you to select the most appropriate practices in Part Three.

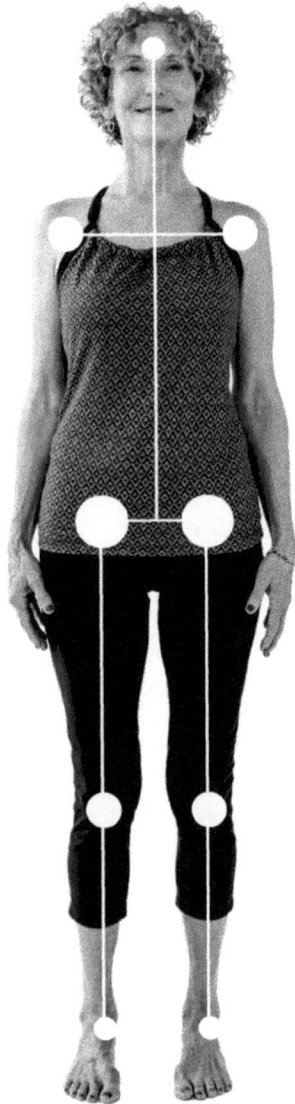

The Blueprint

CHAPTER 7

STRUCTURAL ANATOMY — THE BACKCARE BLUEPRINT

"Everyone is the architect of their own happiness." — *Joseph Pilates*

THE FUNCTION OF THE SPINE

The human body is structured from an exquisite blueprint designed for maximum stability, mobility and expression—all of which occur under the constant weight of gravity.

The human blueprint with its vertical orientation of the spine and legs, and horizontal alignment of the shoulders and hips is brilliant because it minimizes the negative impact of gravity and maximizes freedom.

The spine has several specialized functions: it houses the central nervous system, provides upright orientation which allows for movement across spacial planes. It also serves as a grounding rod for gravity-when the body is properly aligned (which I'll teach you in Part Three).

When proper attention is not paid to alignment and movement the gravitational forces may distort the vertebrae, disrupt the healthy flow of blood and lymph, and impede the neural impulses. Any disruption to this blueprint increases the risk for any number of issues—chronic back pain among them.

With proper alignment, gravitational forces are directed down from the head, through the four curves of the spine, spreading horizontally across the pelvis, grounding down the legs and feet, where it is released into the earth.

With proper alignment you can improve the flow of vital energy through your entire body to heal and create good health.

THE 4 CURVES OF THE SPINE

Your spine has four natural curves that resist gravity's descent and provide mobility and motion. The spinal axis consists of the head, spine, and pelvis. The curves of each section are numbered from top to bottom. For example, L1 is the topmost vertebra of the lumbar spine and L5 is the bottommost vertebra. Let's start with the pelvis and move up the spine.

Pelvis

The pelvis is made from two hip bones (ilium), one sacrum, and one tailbone (coccyx). Although the pelvis as a whole is not counted as one of the curves, the sacrum and tailbone are. The bottom of each ilium bone is shaped to a point—the ischial tuberosity or "sit bones"—which are made for sitting. Two sacroiliac (SI) joints join the sacrum and ilium bones together and are easily located at the back of the pelvic bones, one on each side. The SI joints have a very complex shape with many ridges and rough spots to hold the ilium bones together. Dysfunctional SI joints can cause great pain. This area is a common source of back pain in women who menstruate because hormone fluctuations (increased progesterone) loosen the connective tissue around the sacrum destabilizing the SI joints. In addition, poor posture (such as sitting with one leg crossed over the other or sitting on the sacrum instead of the sit bones) can put uneven weight into these joints.

Sacral Curve (Sacrum/Tailbone)

The sacral curve is part of the pelvis. It is a convex (outward) curve consisting of the sacrum and the coccyx or tailbone. The tailbone (CX1–CX3/5) has three

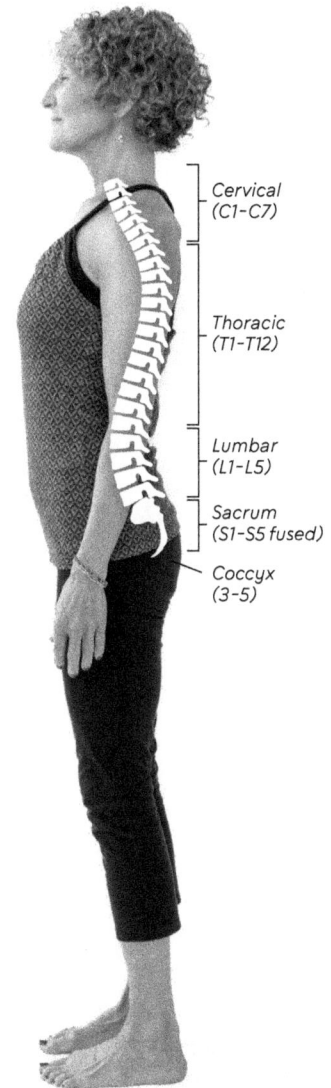

Cervical
(C1-C7)

Thoracic
(T1-T12)

Lumbar
(L1-L5)

Sacrum
(S1-S5 fused)

Coccyx
(3-5)

Pain-Free Posture

> *When the spine is misaligned, gravitational forces increase, causing distortion in the curves of the spine.*

to five fused tiny bones which taper to the bottom and curve inward to the pubic bone. The sacrum is made of five fused vertebrae (S1–S5) that form a diamond-like shape and connect to the top of the tailbone and to both pelvic bones.

Both structures are weight-bearing and integral to walking, standing, and sitting. There is plenty of mobility in the hip sockets to allow for graceful movement. When you walk, one ilium bone rocks forward while the other rocks backward and together the whole pelvis sways side to side. In between them sits the sacrum, designed for stability, not movement. It also rocks forward and backward when you walk—but only a tiny, tiny bit—in a motion called nutation. The swaying movement of the pelvis nourishes your lower back, massaging the entire spine. Too much sitting and too little movement tightens the hips and restricts freedom of motion, while sitting or moving in an asymmetrical pattern puts excess pressure into the SI joints.

Lumbar Curve (Lower Back)

The lumbar curve is concave in shape and comprised of five vertebrae—L1–L5. The lumbar vertebrae are the largest of the spine, providing the most stability and least mobility. Because L5 is 'functionally' fused to S1 and does not move at all, S1–L5 and L5–L4 are common sites of pain and injury. All the vertebrae above L5 can and should be mobile enough to ensure normal and healthy function. Here, the sacral curve changes direction and scoops upwards into the lumbar curve. Unfortunately, the way most people slouch backwards when sitting is both atrocious and dangerous. Sitting on the sacrum instead of the sit bones flattens or reverses the natural inward curve of the lumbar spine and dumps gravity into the vertebrae. Double ouch! Improper sitting is perhaps the biggest cause of chronic back pain.

Thoracic Curve (Upper Back)

The thoracic curve is a convex curve made of twelve vertebrae in the upper back—T1–T12. At the juncture of L1 and T12, the spinal curve again reverses from the inward curve of the lumbar to the outward curve of the thoracic spine. All twelve ribs attach directly to the back of the spine, but only ribs 1–10 connect to the breastbone (sternum) in the front. Ribs 11 and 12 connect only to the back of the spine and float freely in the front, hence their nickname the "floating ribs." These two specialized ribs act like calipers, where they expand on inhalation and retract on exhalation as the ribcage expands and contracts with the breath. The thoracic vertebrae are medium-sized, allowing for greater mobility than the lumbar vertebrae, especially when twisting side to side and when breathing deeply.

Cervical Curve (Neck)

The cervical neck is a concave curve of seven vertebrae (C1–C7). Here the spine changes direction again at the junction of T1–C7, curving inward from the base of your neck up to the base of the skull. These vertebrae are the smallest in size, allowing for the greatest range of movement. Since most of our sense organs are located in the head, it makes sense that the neck would have the most mobility in order to turn the head and locate the sounds, scents, sights and tastes of the world around us. The top two vertebrae of the neck are specialized in their shape and function and called the Atlas (C1) and the Axis (C2).

Skull (Head)

The skull is seated on top of the neck at the atlas-axis junction. The axis (C2) has an upward bony point and the atlas (C1) has an oval shape that rests upon the axis. The head mimics the earth, spinning on an axis. These unique features allow the head to turn, rotate, twist, extend and flex allowing maximum mobility and range of motion. However, the weight of gravity pressing down on the skull, weighing between 8–12 pounds, is enough to cause pain and discomfort in the neck and back.

Together, the design of the two convex and two concave curves allow for maximum range of movement and freedom of expression. A majority of people experience pain where the spine changes direction: where the skull meets the spine (C1–C2), where the base of the neck merges with the thoracic spine (C7–T1), where the base of the thoracic curve becomes the lumbar curve (T12–L1) and where the base of the lumbar curve joins the sacrum (L5–S1).

Is one of these points your hotspot for chronic back pain? Rest assured; you can solve all these issues with the techniques in Part Three. Read on!

SEVEN SPINAL MOVEMENTS

A neutral and balanced spine provides the maximum range of movement and highest freedom of expression. An optimal posture balances all muscles of the body, especially the muscles of the spine. In a neutral position, the forces of gravity are at their lowest, while the flow of blood, lymph, cranial-sacral fluid and energy is at their greatest. In Part Three, I'll show you how to resist gravity, traction your spine, and create optimal posture and healthy flow to significantly reduce or eliminate the back pain.

1. Forward Bend (Spinal Flexion)

A forward bend is a contraction of the belly muscles and extension of the back muscles. This is the most common pattern of movement for all people. When you cradle an infant in your arms, sit a child on your hip, carry a bag of groceries to the kitchen, sit for hours in a vehicle or hunched over a computer, stand at the stove cooking, bend over to vacuum the carpet or to fold laundry, plant flowers, mow the lawn, or weed the garden . . . you are in a spinal flexion. Most of life is a forward bend, so it's vital to learn how to bend forward properly, without underusing, overusing, or misusing your body.

2. Backbend (Spinal Extension)

A backbend or spinal extension is a contraction of back muscles and extension of the belly muscles. I bet you'd never reach for a coffee mug by standing with your back to the cabinet, reaching your arm up over your head and doing a backbend to grab the mug from behind. Although backbends rarely happen during daily life, they are great counter movements for a forward-bending lifestyle and are healthy for the spine. Most everyone would benefit from more spinal extensions.

3. Side Bend to Right (Lateral Flexion)

A side bend or lateral flexion to the right is a contraction of the muscles on the right side of the spine and an extension of the muscles on the left side.

4. Side Bend to Left (Lateral Flexion)

A side bend or lateral flexion to the left is a contraction of the muscles on the left side of the spine and an extension of the muscles on the right.

Stretching both sides is very important as it stretches the intercostal muscles (located between the ribs), invigorating the diaphragm muscles responsible for breathing. Lateral flexion stretches the psoas and quadratus (QL) muscles, preventing the rib cage from being pulled down towards the hips, compressing the lower back and causing strain and pain.

5. Twist to Right (Spinal Rotation)

A spinal rotation or twist combines the extension of the spine with the rotation of the spine. Twisting to the right contracts the muscles on the right side of the spine and stretches the muscles along the left side.

6. Twist to Left (Spinal Rotation)

Twisting to the left contracts the muscles of the left side of the spine and stretches the muscles along the right side.

Spinal rotation done properly is an excellent tonic for the whole spine. Twisting will tone the central nervous system, calming the sympathetic nervous system (fight/flight/freeze response) and stimulating the parasympathetic nervous system (rest/digest/heal). It mobilizes the vertebrae, strengthens the back muscles and moves the cerebrospinal spinal fluid, lubricating the joints of the spine. However, twisting with poor alignment or with a compressed spine can be painful, and many people tweak their back reaching for something in the backseat of their car. Done incorrectly, twisting can impinge on a nerve, pull a muscle, or strain a tendon. Twists can also aggravate SI joint dysfunction and inflamed facet joints, increasing back pain.

7. Spinal Traction (Vertical Extension)

Vertical extension, also known as spinal traction, is a simple process to lengthen the spine along the vertical axis and offset gravitational pressures on the vertebrae, discs

> **Spinal compression is not natural, nor part of the human blueprint.**

and nerves. Vertical extension is not the same as a spinal extension (backbend), nor is it the type of traction you see in a hospital with pulleys and strings that one might need after a bad car accident. This type of traction harnesses balanced muscular action to get the spine out from under the downward forces of gravity. It brings your posture back to neutral alignment consistent with the natural blueprint. Spinal traction also unweights the spinal joints, taking pressure off the nerves and discs. It allows the vertebrae to move back into proper position with one another. It is one of the most important techniques you'll learn in this book and the cornerstone of *The BackCare Blueprint* program. As you gain proficiency with vertical extension and improve spinal alignment, you'll stand taller and prouder, with dignity, poise and grace, without the pain.

SPINAL COMPRESSION

Spinal Compression is not natural, nor part of the human blueprint. It's a collapse of the spine and is the opposite of spinal traction (vertical extension). Compression occurs when you neglect to vertically extend your spine and regularly move in all seven directions. Compression is not one of the seven spinal movements, nor proper spinal alignment, but it is very, very common. Compression results from a combination of the downward gravitational pressure on the spine due to poor postural habits, unbalanced and weak muscles, and inactivity—all of which contribute to chronic back pain. When compression arises, all parts of the vertebral column can be compromised—the spinal cord, cranio-sacral fluid, spinal nerves, nerve roots, discs, facet joints, ligamentum flavum and bony vertebrae.

It is both my experience and opinion that spinal compression is the root cause of most musculoskeletal issues, including herniated discs, nerve impingement, DDD, facet joint dysfunction and SI joint issues, reverse curvature, spondylolisthesis, osteoarthritis, and scoliosis.

In addition, a lack of weight-bearing exercises can diminish bone growth and be detrimental to spinal health.

The seven spinal movements combined with the motion of the arms and legs create an incredible array of gestures with which to express yourself. But to express your uniqueness fully your body needs to be able to move freely. And that reminds me of John. John was a local tree farmer who came to my public yoga classes to address the nagging pain in his lower back. He received a medical diagnosis that revealed a herniated disc at L4–L5, a very common site. The bulge was serious because all of John's work was physically strenuous. Each farm chore he performed, every movement he made, increased the risk of rupturing the disc. So, we added private sessions, where I taught John how to radically improve his alignment to get pressure off the L4–L5 disc and learn to move without pain using the same techniques presented in *The BackCare Blueprint* Program. John's transformation was a beautiful process to observe. He came to me crooked, panicked, and in serious pain. And in just eight weeks, he walked away standing tall, in much less pain, with much more confidence.

A month after his program ended, John called me, elated. "Hey Lynne. Guess what? I kept doing exactly what you told me to do, every day, and it worked! I'm finally off ALL pain-meds and I'm completely free of back pain." Even now, whenever I run into John, he always says, "I'm still following your advice and I'm still free of pain." I'm so proud of him for sticking with the program. Such is the result of the combined power of the Done-With-You and Do-It-Yourself self-care approaches.

Healthy Movement vs Unhealthy Movement

In whichever direction you move—bending forward, backwards, to the right or left, twisting right or left, or extending the spine as you reach overhead—it's essential to establish proper alignment before you move and maintain it while you move,

> *Spinal compression is the root cause of most musculoskeletal issues.*

" —————

*To remedy
spinal
compression,
you must learn
to unweight
your spine
in everyday
postures.*

otherwise you increase the risk of reinjuring your back, yet again. Healthy movement is biomechanically sound. It harnesses the natural levers and fulcrum points of the body's original blueprint and uses them to decrease stress on the joints of the spinal vertebrae. Moving your body in good alignment will always feel free, graceful, and natural. It will ease the pain. Moving with misalignment will feel more strained and restricted. Unfortunately, this will also increase pain. It takes time to relearn patterns of movement, but in my humble opinion, it is not only rewarding, but necessary when faced with chronic back pain resulting from structural misalignment. To remedy spinal compression, you must learn to unweight your spine in everyday postures. And that is one of the first lessons I'll teach you in Part Three. The exercises that follow will help you reorient your habitual postural pattern (cocktail pose), begin to increase range of motion, and cultivate healthy patterns of movement. Remember, I've got your back! Now let's take the next step and learn how the breath can impact chronic back pain.

CHAPTER 8

THE POWER OF BREATH

"Feelings come and go like clouds in a windy sky.
Conscious breathing is my anchor." — *Thich Nhat Hanh*

MODERN EPIDEMIC: UNDER-BREATHING

Far too many people hold their breath. Holding the breath or "under-breathing" is so common that I consider it to be an unrecognized epidemic. This phenomenon exists because most people are not taught to breathe properly, nor to utilize breath to reduce pain and speed healing. Your doctor can't teach you how to breathe consciously, and very few holistic practitioners offer this as a service. The lack of knowledge concerning the use of breath as a tool for healing is another reason I wrote this book. My goal is to show you how you can relieve chronic back pain by incorporating simple breathing techniques into your routine. But before I do, let me tell you about Laura and Marjorie.

Laura came to me with intense pain and tension in her neck. The stiffness and tightness she experienced severely limited her ability to turn her neck from side to side. Her range of motion was only about ten degrees in either direction. Severely limited rotation made driving extremely dangerous because Laura could not turn her head to look over her shoulder and out the window to see beside or behind her. Rightly so, she was afraid of getting into a car accident. When we first met, I immediately noticed that Laura was barely breathing. Both stiffness and fear caused her to hold her breath in, so I began by teaching Laura a simple exercise to realign her feet, and for the first time in a long time, she started drinking in deeper breaths. From there, we worked on correcting the alignment of her upper back and shoulder girdle. After a few weeks, her neck mobility significantly improved, and after twelve weeks, was fully restored. Laura was delighted that she could turn her head a full 180 degrees from right to left and back without any stiffness or pain and her confidence to drive safely returned.

Marjorie's story is similar. She sought my help to address unbearable tension in her lower back and sacrum which occurred from long hours seated at her computer, editing video footage. Again, the first thing I noticed was how Marjorie also held her breath. I guided her through one of my favorite breathing techniques, and during the session the pain completely disappeared. Marjorie was amazed that she could feel so good, so quickly. We subsequently worked on her sitting posture so she could continue to breathe freely. Marjorie went back to work editing films, but this time without discomfort or tension.

The journey that both Laura and Marjorie took to relieve their back pain was one that involved moving from autonomic breath to conscious breath, and it's important to understand the difference between the two.

THE AUTONOMIC BREATH:
UNCONSCIOUS BREATHING ON AUTOPILOT

Using breath to heal pain may sound foreign to you, but seeing as how you're still alive, it shouldn't. Autonomic breathing is automatic, instinctive, and unconscious. The autonomic breath is what 95% of people default to 95% of the time. It's like breathing with an autopilot setting. While you're busy running your life, "something" is busy breathing for you! Call that brain power or Spirit, either way it's easy to ignore because it can function without your attention. The autonomic breath gets triggered when something disturbing happens, such as the unexpected metallic boom of a dump truck smashing over a pothole, the agonizing cry of a child who trips, falls, and bumps his head, or the flashing lights and wild sirens of an ambulance whizzing by. Any sudden move, sound, or sight that surprises or frightens you will make you gasp and hold your breath! How about that embarrassing moment when you burn your tongue on hot food or your finger on an open flame? Instinct causes you to pant rapidly through the mouth, to extinguish the "fire" or to blow gently on a wound to soothe it. What about that moment when your spouse tells the same story for the millionth time, and you sigh gently with control and discretion so as not to reveal your boredom or disapproval? These normal responses are part of the central nervous system's instinctive mechanism to pull you away from danger and ensure your survival.

Animals never hold their breath a moment longer than danger is present. I've lived with cats for forty years and I know with certainty, a sudden sound or movement will make them jump, but AS SOON AS that stimulation dissolves, the cat relaxes back into its normal "pre-shock" state. Not so with humans! Ever notice yourself, still holding your breath long after a sudden surprise or shock has ended? Even weeks later! Do you know someone who looks as if he or she hasn't exhaled in over a decade? We all have habitual breathing patterns, but holding one's breath is so common it's become a familiar cultural norm. What personal examples come to mind? How does your own breath automatically assist to mitigate an unpleasant situation or soothe a wound? In each circumstance, your body acts to expel pain and heal the injury without you even thinking about it. Rest assured, automatically holding your breath is a pattern that can and must be shifted to conscious breathing for better health.

> ❝
>
> *We all have habitual breathing patterns; holding one's breath is so common it's become a familiar cultural norm.*

> **Breathe with mindfulness and purpose.**

THE CONSCIOUS BREATH:
BREATHING WITH PURPOSE AND AWARENESS

What you must consider next is key! The breath not only carries oxygen into your lungs and bloodstream, but it also carries something sublime, intrinsic, unseen and unappreciated: the life force. Chi, Qi, Ki, Prana, God, Breath of Life, and Holy Spirit are all synonymous for the breath. Breath carries THE animating force, a power without which you'd die. Humans can survive thirty days without food, fourteen days without water, but only a few minutes without the breath. If you stop breathing for four minutes, you'll suffer permanent brain damage. Yes, you'd die from a lack of oxygen, but you also die because the Spirit leaves your body. Between a babies' first breath and a seniors' last breath is life. And breath nourishes your life every step of the way. Breath is the bridge between Spirit and matter, between soul and body.

As you pay attention to your breath and recognize its healing power, you'll begin to breathe with mindfulness and purpose. When you consciously notice your breath pattern in any given moment and how breath reacts to stimulation from the world around you, you can shift from an unconscious breath to a conscious deliberate breath, accessing the power of the life force—the power of the breath to heal. In Part Three, you'll learn to use your breath to reduce back pain. But before we do that, let's do something equally important!

CHAPTER 9

VISION OF HEALTH

"Doctors won't make you healthy. Nutritionists won't make you slim. Teachers won't make you smart. Gurus won't make you calm. Mentors won't make you rich. Trainers won't make you fit. Ultimately, you have to take responsibility to save yourself." — *Naval Ravikant*

To make the shift from expecting others to fix you (DFY) to healing yourself (DIY), you must create a personal Vision of Health. Of all the concepts and techniques I can offer, the formulation of a unique vision of health tops the list. Deep within you already resides everything you could ever desire—health, wealth, and happiness. You just need to focus your awareness and rediscover the place that is already whole and never in pain. As you unearth this treasure within, you'll discover a valuable gem—one that will remind you why you bought this book in the first place. What you discover in creating a Vision of Health will keep you inspired and motivated as you learn some new habits.

YOUR VISION OF HEALTH

This is the very first step I require of all my clients. Often, it's the most challenging step because people who've been locked into a cycle of chronic pain for years have often forgotten what wellness feels like. Knowing exactly what you want to do, how you wish to feel, and exactly what health looks like—to you—will be your guiding compass. Once you have created a basic vision of health, you may clarify or embellish it over time. Return to your vision every day and use it as motivation to stay on track with your new pain-free practices!

To Begin

Right now, take a comfortable seated position or stand upright. Gradually, turn your attention away from thoughts and problems and place it fully on the breath. Notice the length of your inhale and exhale and begin to breathe more deeply. Breathe steadily in and steadily out without holding your breath. It's important not to strain. Allow yourself to drop down out of your head and settle into your physical body. Allow yourself to be present in this moment. Let go of thoughts, let go of sensations, let go of doing anything. Imagine dropping down into a quiet, calm, beautiful place within yourself, and enter your very own sacred space. Sacred space is the awareness of unlimited possibility, unbounded choice, and infinite options and total freedom. Ifs, ands, buts, can'ts and don'ts do not exist here. In sacred space, you give yourself permission to create whatever you wish, just because you are special, precious, and completely deserving of your dreams.

Now, in your quiet space, imagine yourself fully alive, fully healed. Stay positive and picture yourself fully healed, fully alive . . . because in sacred space you are!!

Keep breathing gently, steadily in and out.

Notice the following:

·   Where are you? What are you doing?

·   Are you with others or by yourself?

·   What clothes are you wearing?

·   What's the expression on your face?

·   How does your body feel?

·   How does your heart feel? What emotions are present?

·   What thoughts pass through your mind?

Paint a bright picture of total health. Be as specific as you can, creating a powerful vision of health. Engage all of your senses: allowing pictures, colors, sounds, feelings, to arise without censorship. Imagine yourself as healthy, see yourself as healthy, feel yourself as healthy, taste yourself as healthy, smell yourself as healthy, hear yourself as healthy, touch yourself as healthy. Spend several minutes creating your unlimited vision of health. When you feel complete with this meditation, slowly open your eyes.

Write down your vision of health, before it fades away.

Use positive, affirmative, descriptive first-person language.

66

Each morning, starting tomorrow, review your personal vision of health.

_____

_____

_____

_____

_____

Each morning, starting tomorrow, review your personal vision of health. The more time you spend refining your vision, the clearer it will become, and in this process, you learn to retrain your brain. Make this a daily ritual, one where you tune into the part of you that is healthy and always feels amazing.

PART TWO CONCLUSION

So, let's recap Part Two. A chronically misaligned spine can have negative consequences. It can cause many issues, from DDD, to arthritis, disc herniation, stenosis, and beyond. Poor posture disrupts the natural physical blueprint and diminishes your capacity to breathe, and sets off a chain of events that can lead to chronic back pain. When body and breath are constantly out of sync, structural misalignments become embedded in the body, resulting in habitually chronic patterns that lead to chronic pain. Fortunately, the good news is that you can alter your habits and change your patterns. Each time you adjust your mindset, realign your spine, harness your breath, and correct structural misalignments by yourself, you supplant healthier habits that reduce back pain and increase joy!

Why, just by reading Part Two, you've quantumly upgraded your knowledge. If you have considered a new attitude (pain is my friend, not my enemy), discovered newfound objectivity ("the" pain instead of "my" pain), contemplated a new belief (Yes, I can heal) and accepted a new strategy (Done-With-You, instead of Done-For-You), then you've already become a more willing participant in your healing process. And in doing so, you've received valuable information and learned something new about yourself. By identifying your "cocktail pose" and examining the four spinal curves, you can start to make connections between the types of pain you frequently experience with associated tissues, injuries, and possible causes.

You've read how pain sends you messages and gives you clues about the cause of chronic back pain so that you can heal, and now you understand why communicating with pain is better than medicating it. Perhaps you can see the most common structural issues causing your back pain. The vision of health you've created as a guiding compass, combined with deep self-inquiry will help you properly apply the techniques in Part Three. Look how far you've come!! Well done.

Now it's time to learn the specific alignment techniques and pain-free practices that will help you reduce or eliminate chronic back pain without any medical intervention.

PAIN-FREE PRACTICES TO HEAL YOUR BACK

In Part Three, I'll provide specific instructions for optimizing your posture and harnessing the healing power of your breath. You'll learn how to build better alignment from the ground up—from the feet to the head—in the everyday positions of standing, sitting, walking, bending and twisting since those are the movements you do most of the time. Adjusting your daily posture will have the greatest impact and benefit on the health of your spine, because the health of your spine determines how young you feel.

Before you start any practice, please consider your recent level of activity.

Have you been too sedentary, moving too little? Have you moved too much and strained or overexerted your muscles? Or have you misused or mistreated your back? With this understanding, you can choose specific practices to help balance your habitual tendencies. Every time you move, you do so under the effects of gravity, so let's take a look at how gravity impacts your spine, potentially causing back pain.

CHAPTER 10

HARNESS GRAVITY TO HEAL YOUR SPINE

"The natural healing force within each one of us is the greatest force in getting well."
— *Hippocrates*

Gravity can negatively impact a physical misalignment, putting more pressure into the weak area of your spine and thereby increasing physical pain. Think about the four spinal curves. From the delicate cervical bones to the large stable lumbar bones, these vertebrae are designed to channel the forces of gravity from your head, down your legs and feet, and into the earth. When posture is optimal, there is much less gravitational pressure on your spine, especially on the lower back. When posture is misaligned or lacking integrity, your body will be more subject to the pressure of gravity pushing down on you.

In order to reduce back pain, it's imperative to push back against gravity, and create and sustain optimal posture. One way to do this is to make a constant connection between the earth beneath you and the space above you. In this chapter, you'll learn three specific techniques that will help you get out from under the weight of gravity, significantly reduce back pain, and put you on the road back to health.

KINETIC AWARENESS

Kinetic Awareness (KA) harnesses the passive power of gravity to reduce muscular and fascial tension. This technique can help in situations of underuse, overuse and misuse. KA provides immediate feedback about the condition of your back muscles and fascia because the weight of your body resting on the balls will reveal areas of soreness, tension, knots—as well as healthy tissue. It's a wonderful "Do-It-Yourself" method to increase awareness and relieve tension in the back.

I first encountered the KA method in a weekend workshop. A group of forty students spent the entire time laying on the floor and slowly, methodically rolling out every part of the body with various sized rubber, foam, air-filled, and spongy balls. Imagine spending three hours rolling two balls down the length of your spine; a span of only 2–3 feet depending on your height. It was a revelatory process which heightened my awareness of the mind-body connection and, more importantly, the condition of my spine. I was able to locate spots of muscle tension and soft tissue tenderness. I noticed a difference between the right and left sides of my back. (You'll understand exactly what I mean when you try this). The ball-rolling made my back feel elastic and free. The lasting effects were so incredible I decided to introduce all my students and clients to "ball work" or KA.

Before you can practice, you'll need to purchase several pairs of balls of varying size from 1" to 6". The balls I use most often range from 2"–3". Tennis balls (preferably used ones) are easy to find and you may already have some. If so, start the KA practice today. The pinky and rainbow brand solid rubber balls are a little smaller and softer than tennis balls, which makes the initial experience less intense. For an average-sized person, all three types are excellent choices and can be used interchangeably to roll out your back. You can find the pinky balls, rainbow balls and others in toy stores, pet stores, big box stores, and online fitness shops.

Kinetic Awareness is a wonderful way to uncover and unbind hidden pockets of tension in your whole body—especially in the muscles alongside your spine. The KA process takes you on a journey deep into your body—where you're able to witness tension at the gross level of the bulk of a muscle to the more subtle level of small muscle bundles, and finally the most subtle level of individual muscle fibers. More than anything—this process taught me to face physical "pain" instead of resisting or running away from it.

Before you begin KA, I will be honest. There were times during the workshop when the physical sensation (pain) was just too intense for me to stay in one spot and breathe deeply. The first few times you roll out your spine you might also encounter intense pain. If you do, don't give up. Don't decide ball work won't work . . . because it does, and it will. Almost everyone in the workshop encountered a "hotspot" where sensation was just too strong for them to bear. Most of my students and clients had an aversion to KA the first few times they tried it. This initial experience is very

> 66
>
> *Kinetic Awareness is a wonderful way to uncover and unbind hidden pockets of tension in your whole body— especially in the muscles alongside your spine.*

> *Remain still and observe with great curiosity where you hold tension.*

common. So, don't spend any time on the spots that are too painful for you. Roll as close to them as you can, and then skip over them, or use a softer ball. There is always tomorrow! Eventually, the hotspots will dissolve, and you'll be able to roll out your entire spine without pain and with great joy. Everyone I've taught KA to falls in love with it after a few tries. I'm certain you will, too!

Pain-Free Practice #1: Roll Away Back Pain

(Photo sequence on following pages.) Once you have at least one pair of balls, it's time to begin. Make sure to wear a tight-fitting shirt without extra layers (loose fabric tends to bunch up around the balls as you roll). Lay down on a carpet or yoga mat instead of a wood floor, as the balls tend to slip out from underneath on a smooth surface. Bend your knees and place your feet flat on the floor and parallel to your hips. Lift your head and place the two balls, touching, under the C7/T1 vertebrae (the big bone at the base of your neck). Rest your upper back down onto the balls. Lift and hold your arms up in front of your head with elbows bent and hands in prayer position. This arm position makes space between your shoulder blades for the balls to fit nicely without excess pressure. Use this position as you roll the upper back from the neck to the base of the shoulder blades. Once the balls are below the shoulder blades and on the mid-back, you can rest your arms on your belly or on the floor.

Once you are on the first spot (C7/T1), remain still and observe with great curiosity where you hold tension, how you react to that tension, and what emotions or thoughts arise from the weight of your back on the balls. Notice what happens to the breath as you move towards or onto a tender area. Do you hold your breath? Do you pant rapidly to avert pain? Do you squint your eyes, clench your jaw or fists, or contract other parts of your body in resistance to the sensation?

After thirty seconds, press gently into your feet and roll down next to the second (T1/T2) vertebrae. Again, pause and observe your reactions. After another thirty seconds, roll down to the next vertebrae (T2/T3). Proceed slowly, rolling all the way down your spine, and pausing, observing, breathing, watching and waiting for tension to dissolve at each vertebra. When you reach the sacrum, do the same. Then, lift your hips enough to separate the balls just a little, and pause, observe, breathe, and repeat—each time widening the balls, until you reach the outer hips. Now you've just finished the "first pass."

If you have time, start over and repeat the entire process two more times, resting between each vertebra for thirty seconds. The physical sensation should be less intense each time. After the "third pass" is complete, do one more—this time gently rolling the balls back and forth over any spot you choose. This rolling technique is especially useful if you find a spot where the muscles are very tight, hard or thick. If there is a band of several muscles in one area that feel equally tight you can roll gently over the entire area just make sure to breathe deeply instead of holding your breath. Remember, the deepest release comes from staying in one spot and breathing deeply while letting go of whatever you are holding.

I want to emphasize the importance of breathing in KA. Every time you exhale, purposefully relax your back muscles. Imagine your spine softening around the balls and tension melting off your back carrying pain and sensation away with it. Every time you inhale, imagine prana, the healing energy or life force, fueling your body and soothing your spine. In this way, breathing becomes a mechanism for releasing pain and increasing wellbeing. To roll out your entire spine three or four times in this manner can take a half hour depending on how quickly or slowly you proceed, and that is determined by how intense or mild the sensations feel.

Again, I cannot overemphasize how important it is to roll past any excruciating spots and rest in areas where you can bear sensation. Every time you roll, roll out your entire spine! Rest on each spot for a minimum of thirty seconds, breathing deeply and being

> *Every time you exhale, purposefully relax your back muscles.*

present, as this is how long it takes for the muscles to release. That being said, once you feel comfortable with this process, you can move a little closer to the tender spots, eventually getting right into them, rolling over every part of your back without skipping a section. If you always skip over the same hotspot, and continually run from pain, you won't receive the full benefits of KA ball work. A big part of this process is to locate pain, meet pain, and release pain.

Note: If you have severe degenerative disk disease or advanced osteoporosis and cannot put the full weight of your body onto the balls without risking damage to the vertebrae, (or you cannot get down onto the floor), you can practice this technique standing against a wall. Here you'll want to start with bent knees so you can use your legs to roll over the balls. This adaptation may be a little awkward, but it's better than nothing.

What a blessed self-care modality KA truly is! I use it every day to maintain spinal health. The cost to get started is minimal, and once you've purchased a few balls, it is completely free. KA can reduce your reliance on massage, chiropractic, and acupuncture care. It will save you money and time driving to and from appointments and reduce the need for painkillers. It will deepen your self-awareness, self-connection and self-appreciation. I hope you fall in love with KA ball work. Please use it daily to take back your health and create relaxation and freedom for yourself. Why, you might find this practice is the only one you need to relieve a sore back!

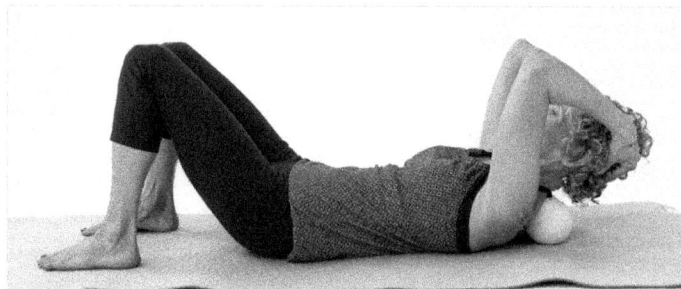

①

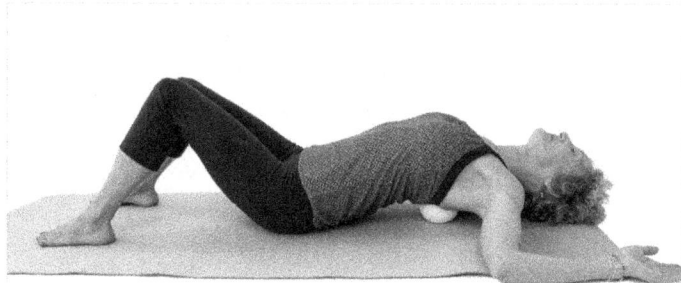

④

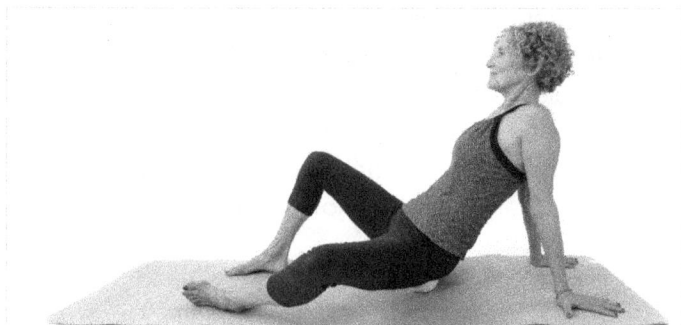

⑦

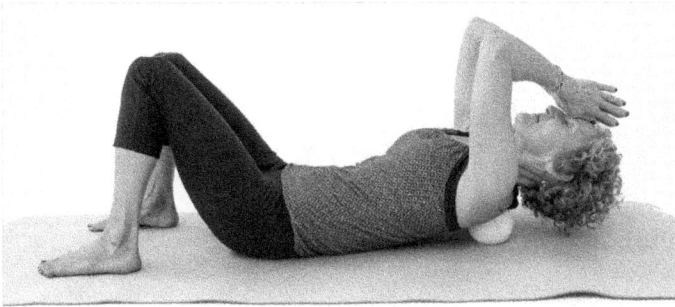

②

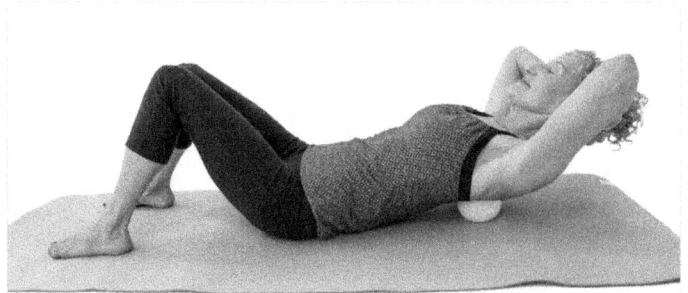

③

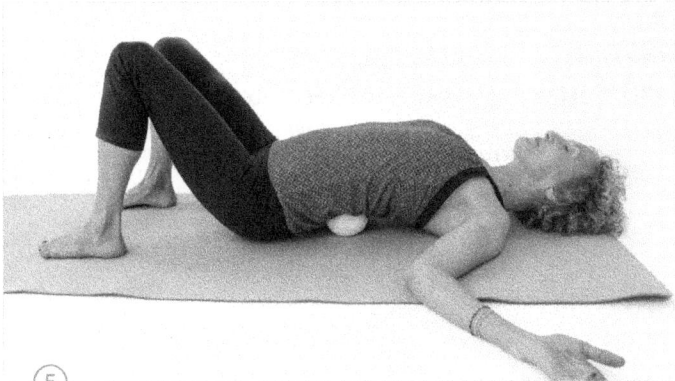

⑤

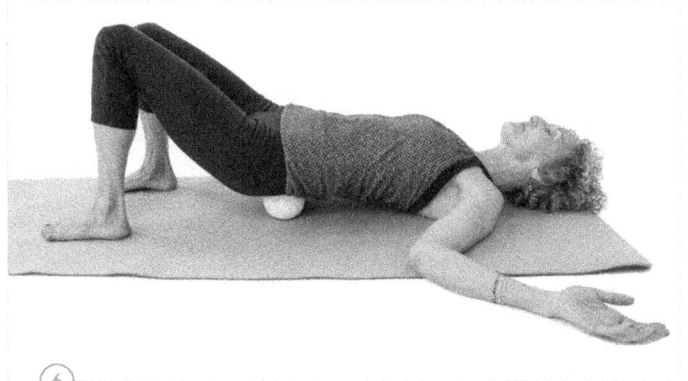

⑥

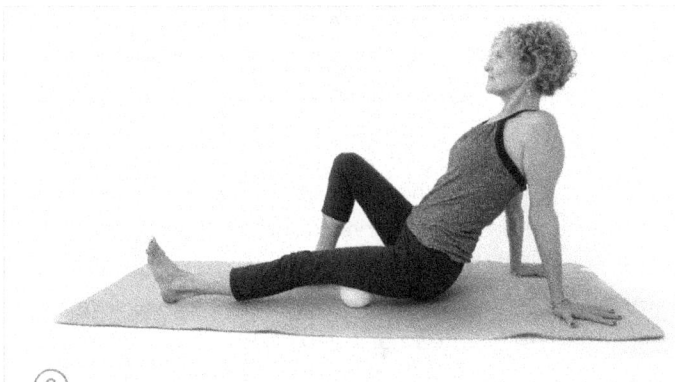

⑧

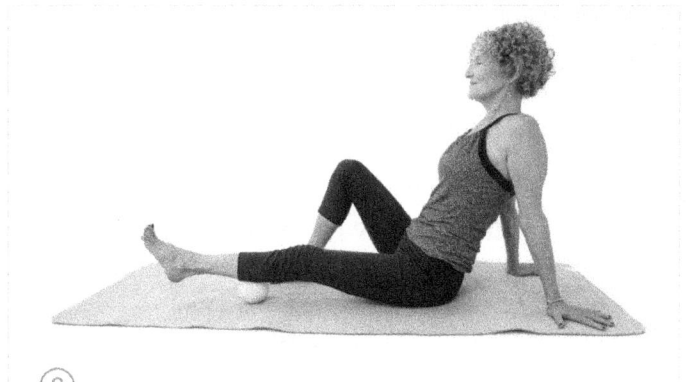

⑨

Pain-Free Practice #2: The Cranio-Cradle Resting Pose

I learned this technique from my cranio-sacral therapist, and it has been a lifesaver in times of extreme duress when my nervous system was triggered and would not calm down. I wish I knew about this simple technique when I suffered from sciatic and lower back pain decades ago, but I'm sure glad I know about it today.

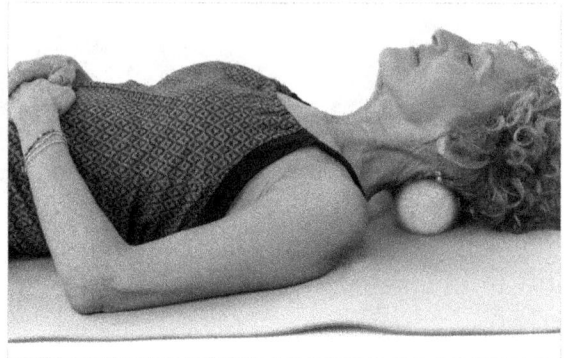

To make the cranio-cradle, you'll need two balls of the same size. Place them both into the toe area of a clean shin or knee length sock and tie off the end so the balls don't slide. Lay down on your back, placing a blanket roll under the backs of your knees if you have any lower back discomfort. Lift your head and place the sock under the base of your skull. The exact position is important, and you have to feel for the sweet spot. To locate this position, rub the fingers of both hands up from the sides of the neck to the base of the skull (occiput), where you'll feel the curve of the skull on both sides. Now move your fingers up and over the curve to the flat area. This is where you want to place the balls.

Once you are resting on the balls, if you haven't found the sweet spot, you can shift position slightly by raising or lowering your chin. A correct position feels comfortable on your skull, an incorrect position will cause the sock ball to pop out from underneath your head. If that keeps happening, place a little cloth under your neck to keep the sock ball in place.

Now that you've found the right spot. Breathe slowly and relax your whole body. Allow the muscles of your face and neck to soften and unwind. Let go of your thoughts. In a few minutes, this position will calm the central nervous system, quiet the mind, release tension in the body—all which help to reduce pain, naturally. Rest quietly until your body tells you it's time to end this practice.

When done correctly, this practice is magic! Pressure on this spot switches the central nervous system from fight/flight/freeze mode to rest/digest/repair mode, supporting vagal nerve function. I've found that it consistently interrupts the endless stream of mental activity which exacerbates pain. More importantly, it activates a state of refined awareness—called the "witness" or "observer" state—which feels like a deep meditative or suspended state of animation where you simply float in an ocean of awareness.

Pain-Free Practice #3: Self-Traction Your Spine

This practical technique is the backbone of *The BackCare Blueprint* program. Learning to self-traction your own spine while standing and sitting is one of the most beneficial techniques you can learn to get yourself out of pain and to keep yourself out of pain. It's a total shock to me that so few health care practitioners teach it to their clients. This technique might be the most helpful one for you and might be the only practice you need to dissolve back pain. In this chapter, I'll explain the key concepts then give you specific instructions to make the most of this simple practice.

First, I'll explain how to decompress the discs and vertebrae using the same technique but with four different arm positions. I suggest you try each position each time you practice. Later, you can combine this self-traction technique with the instructions for standing tall, which I'll cover soon. When you discover the specific arm position that gives you the most relief, please use it every day. If that one becomes less effective, try another.

So, let's begin:

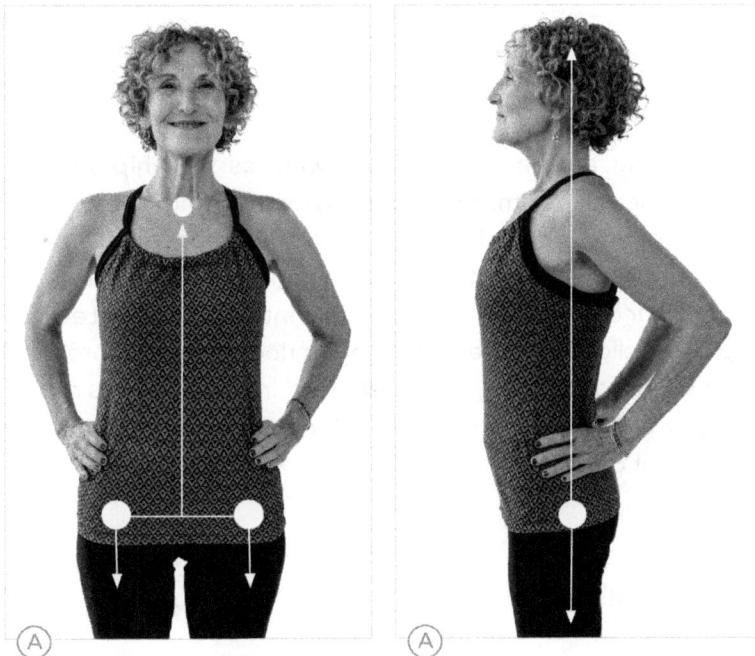

A. Hands on Hips

Stand with your legs parallel and feet as wide as your hip sockets. Breathe deeply. Place your hands on the top of your hips, one on each side. Take a few deep breaths in and out. With the next inhalation, press both hands down onto your hip bones and lift up through your chest. Pull your elbows back slightly so they are a little behind your body. Keep your chest lifted as you breathe in and out. Stay for one minute, and release. Repeat as often as needed throughout the day.

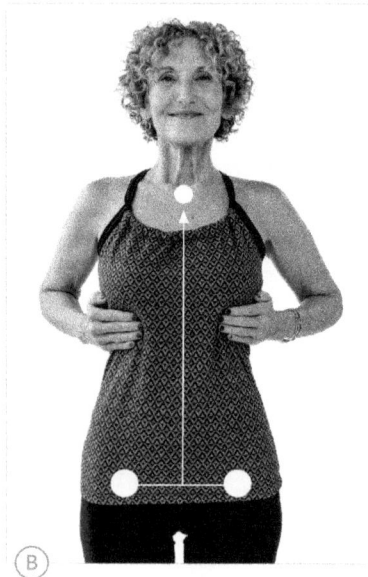

B. Hands on Side of Ribcage

Stand with your feet and legs parallel, as wide as your hip sockets. Breathe deeply. Place your hands—with eight fingers facing forward and thumbs pointing backwards—on the sides of your ribcage (If your hands don't stretch that far, point all ten fingers forward). Take a few deep breaths in and out. With the next inhalation, use both hands to lift your chest up away from your hips. Pull your elbows back slightly so they are a little behind your body. Keep lifting your chest with your hands as you breathe in and out. Stay for one minute, and release. Repeat as often as needed throughout the day.

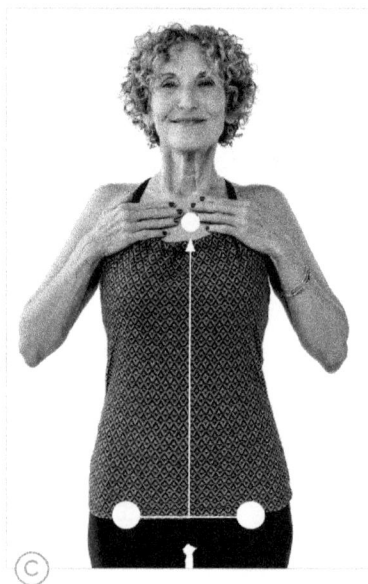

C. Hands on Top of Chest

Stand with your feet and legs parallel, as wide as your hip sockets. Breathe deeply. Place the palms of your hands (with all fingers touching) on the top front of your chest, just below the collar bones. Take a few deep breaths in and out. With the next inhalation, press both palms gently down on your chest and lift your chest up into your hands. Let your elbows drop down slightly so they point to the floor. Keep the pressure of your palms steady and keep your chest lifted into your hands as you breathe in and out. Stay for one minute, and release. Repeat as often as needed throughout the day.

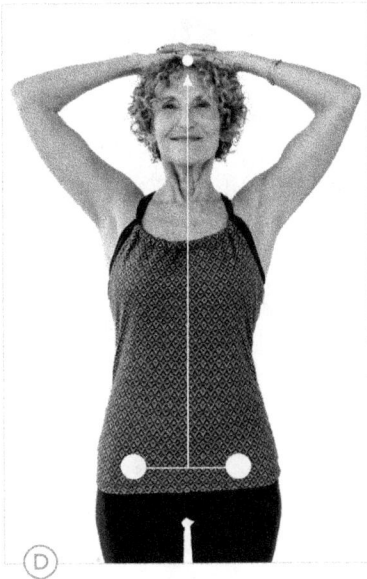

D. Hands on Top of Head

Stand with your feet and legs parallel, as wide as your hip sockets. Breathe deeply. Place one hand on the top of your head, place the second hand on top of the first. Keep your elbows pointing forward, not out to the sides. Take a few deep breaths in and out. With the next inhale, press both palms gently down on top of your head, and as you inhale, simultaneously lift your chest up, towards and into your hands. This will help you lengthen the spine from the lower back through the neck and head. Keep the pressure of your palms steady, your spine tall and chest lifted as you breathe in and out. Stay for one minute, and release. Repeat as often as needed throughout the day.

Each of these variations of spinal self-traction will lengthen the spine, and engage your abdominal and back muscles, creating much needed space along the spinal axis and between the vertebrae. Do your best to lift your chest evenly on all sides (more details on that later) so you don't end up over-tightening your back muscles. After all, you just finished the KA back rolling technique in order to soften the back muscles and make this self-traction exercise easier and more effective.

Pain-Free Practice #4: Ground to Grow

Here's another easy exercise to decompress your own spine and ward off the detrimental effects that gravitational pressure constantly puts on the vertebrae. It's similar to the self-traction exercise, but it's more dynamic because you add the power of the legs and lower body. Here, you'll engage the legs and core muscles to harness the rooting power of the legs, and extend the spine upward (as in the last exercise) to unweight the vertebrae and discs and mitigate the negative effects of gravity. I learned this valuable principle after decades of yoga training. I like to call it "ground to grow." The basic idea is that your body is the bridge between earth and sky. When you learn to actively ground the gravitational forces down into the earth and extend your spine upward towards the sky, you can release pressure in the discs, nerves, and bones of your spine and reduce pain in your back. Less compression equals less pain. Ground to Grow harnesses the equal and opposite actions of the body in relationship to gravity and creates structural balance with integrity. It's the way we connect the lower body with the upper body and it's the best way to "push back" against gravity's downward force. Once you get the hang of this new alignment, you'll be able to ground gravity down your legs into the earth and extend the length of your spine from your hips to your head wherever you go! This will quickly decompress your lower back and give you instant relief.

Let's learn how to decompress your own spine with the "ground to grow" technique. This technique integrates the fourth-hand position (hands on top of head) with the strength of the legs.

To begin:

Stand upright with your feet and legs hip-width apart and parallel (the most stable stance). Place your hands on the very top of your head and interlace all ten fingers. Firmly, yet gently, press both hands down onto your head. Imagine you're standing at the end of a diving board. Take a big breath in and bend your knees. As you exhale, straighten your legs by pressing from your hips straight down through your legs and feet into the floor (as you would push down on a diving board). As your legs straighten, extend your

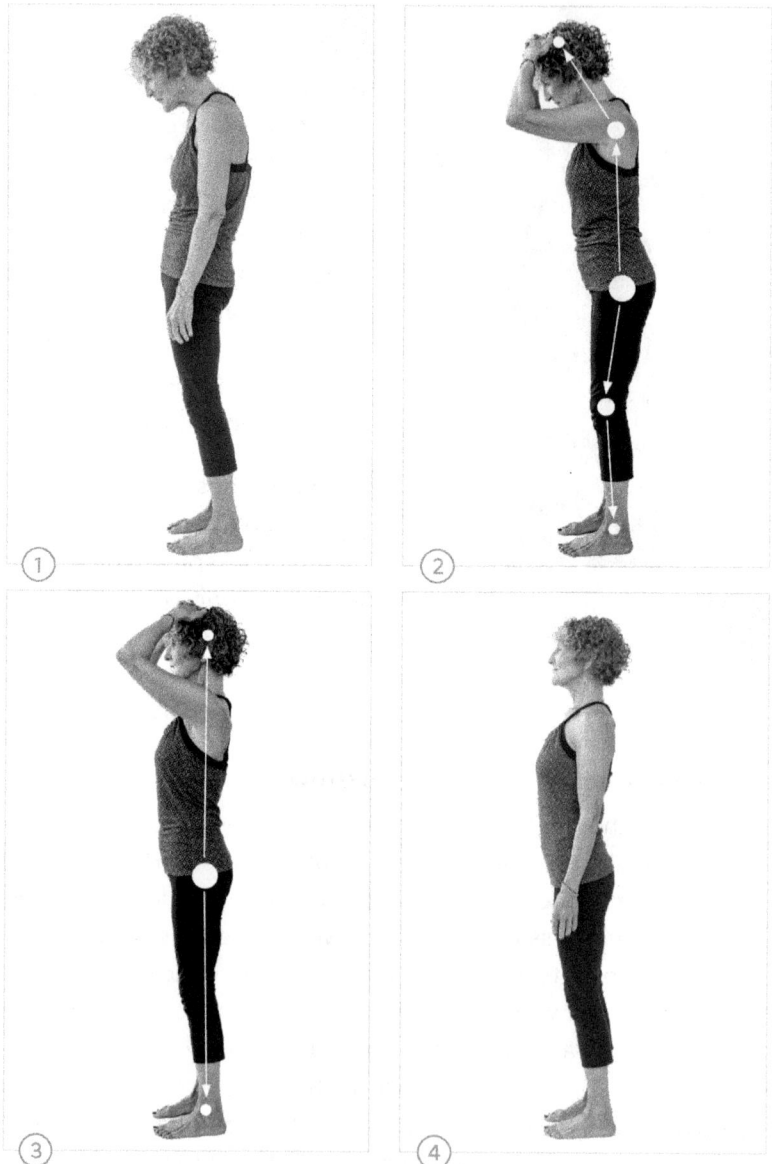

Ground to Grow

whole spine upward into your hands. Feel your spine lengthen and grow. Repeat as many times as it takes for you to feel the action of "ground to grow." As this exercise becomes familiar, you'll find you can both ground and grow simultaneously.

Done properly, this exercise will give you an immediate way to lengthen your spine and resist the force of gravity. At the apex of this movement, your body will feel integrated with strong calves and quadriceps, toned abdominals, extended spine and neck that support the weight of the head. Once you've got the hang of it, at the top of your fullest extension, lower your hands down by your hips and maintain the stance. This is a simple mountain pose! Do you feel as strong as a mountain?

Unweighting the spine is an integral part of *The BackCare Blueprint* book and online video program because structural integrity is what breaks the vicious cycle of misalignment and chronic pain. Now you have four excellent ways to help yourself unweight your aching spine: KA Ball Rolling, Cranio-Cradle, Self-Traction, and Ground to Grow. I recommend you do these exercises at least once every day. You can use the self-traction method during the day as often as you need to reduce pain. I promise, it will make a big difference!!

CHAPTER 11

EFFECTIVE ALIGNMENT FOR PAIN-FREE POSTURE

"Health is a vehicle, not a destination." — *Joshua Fields Millburn*

In order to eliminate back pain, you may need a total postural alignment makeover. To give your spine the support it needs to transform your 'cocktail pose' into a pain-free posture, you'll need to shore up your entire body. To accomplish that, I'll teach you the basics of optimal alignment, aka the science of biomechanics. Once you understand the basics, you can apply the exact same alignment to any activity— sitting, standing, walking, running, biking, skiing, hiking, sleeping—you name it! These biomechanical alignments are universal to every human body. They are the template or blueprint for healthy movement. Since your body is designed to move with ease and grace in order to express yourself fully, it makes sense to align your body properly. Within this human blueprint, one process is a constant—your legs and lower body should support your spine and upper body. Once you understand this, adjusting your alignment becomes simpler.

In this section, let's consider the two halves of the body—the lower body and the upper body—and the way they function, together, to create optimal alignment. The feet, shins, thighs, and pelvis make up the lower body and the spine, neck, head, shoulders, arms and hands comprise the upper body. For anyone with back pain, especially for people with low back pain, the connection between the lower body and upper body is extremely important. When you use the lower body to ground the force of gravity into the earth, you can create more support for the upper body. The entire length of the spine is designed to rise upward from the earth so you can enjoy mobility of the vertebrae and freedom across all seven types of spinal movement (which I explained in chapter seven).

> **Within this human blueprint, one process is a constant—your legs and lower body should support your spine and upper body.**

While making any structural adjustment (or when moving in general), it is necessary to breathe deeply and steadily—especially while you are practicing new postural habits. When the body is way out of alignment, it's prudent to make gradual movements towards optimal alignment. If you make an adjustment and experience a sharp pain or more discomfort, you might have moved too far or too fast trying to shift from your habitual posture towards an aligned one. Realigning the muscles and bones does require effort, but you never want to force your body into a position. Done correctly, the effort you make to properly align will stay in the muscles and will make the joints feel better, not worse. This delicate balance is hard to adequately convey in a book, so please take a look at *The BackCare Blueprint* online video program, too. And of course, do reach out to me for individual support if you get stuck. You can find my contact information in the resource section.

Whenever I teach alignment, I always start by adjusting the feet and working up the body. It's important to know that weak or misaligned feet and legs cannot adequately support a healthy spine, while strong, optimally aligned legs can and do. In fact, it's been said that the legs "govern the spine," so it's essential to start at ground level.

Since gravity always pushes down on your body, thereby compressing your spine, you'll need to build a strong stance from the ground up. And since it's your feet that touch the earth, it's good to set the foundation of your feet first because any misalignment in the feet can create misalignment in any of the joints (knees, hips, spine, neck, shoulders) higher up. Aligning the feet will improve your whole posture.

We'll combine the alignment of the upper and lower body to create an integrated, structurally sound standing posture. Voila! Soon you'll know how to shift your "cocktail pose" into pain-free poses while standing, sitting, walking, bending and twisting. Finally, I suggest you use a mirror for visual feedback as you learn to adjust

> **When the body is way out of alignment, it's prudent to make gradual movements towards optimal alignment.**

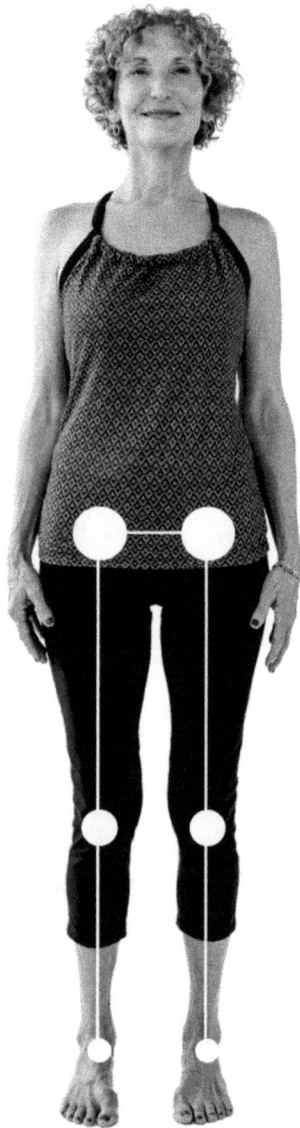

Ground to Grow

your posture. It will help you see your patterns more clearly, know when you are "in or out" of alignment, and recognize what each feels like. Typically, an out of whack position will hurt and a correct position will feel neutral or even good. In the beginning, the optimal position might feel unfamiliar or foreign, because you are used to the way your body feels when chronically misaligned. Let me assure you, with time and practice you will come to know the difference between the two. Then, you can consciously choose the new pain-free alignment instead of the old pain-causing habits.

GROUND TO GROW

Standing: Align the Lower Body (Ground)

In order to properly support the spine you must precisely align the lower body first. The overall aim here is to stack the joints of the lower body—feet, ankles, knees—in a vertical line directly beneath the hip sockets to create a strong and easeful stance. Practice this alignment in bare feet, so you can tune into the feeling of your feet, toes and arches.

Let's identify a few important markers so you can align properly:

· second toe

· center of ankle

· middle of heel

· center of knee

· hip socket

· front of the pelvis

1. Align the Feet with the Hips

To stand correctly, your feet must be placed as wide as your hip sockets, and parallel to one another. To find "hips distance apart," you need to locate your hip sockets or the anterior superior iliac spine (ASIS), anatomical jargon for the top front part of your hip bones. Place your fingertips on the front of your pelvis and feel around to locate the most forward-pointing bones (one on each side), located right above the hip sockets. Now, bend over and press gently on the front of your ankles to locate the soft spot between the two main tendons. This is the center of the ankle. Stand back up and look down your legs, adjusting each foot so the center of the ankle lines up with the center of the hip socket (ASIS). Congratulations, you have just set your feet "hips distance apart."

Now, set both feet parallel. To do this, look down at your feet and notice in which direction they point—straight forward, outwards (duck toe), or inwards (pigeon toe). If both feet do not point straight forward, you'll need to adjust them so they do. Line up the base of your second toes with the center of the ankles, lining up the center of the heel (where the Achilles tendon attaches) with both the center of the ankle and second toe. Well done! Both feet should now be parallel and symmetrical.

It's also important to correct fallen arches (pronated feet). To do this, lift and spread all ten toes. You'll feel the arches of your feet lift, too. Now balance the weight on the four corners of the feet: big toe mound, inner heel, little toe mound, and outer heel. These four points of contact with the earth are important and must be equally weighted to properly support your spine. To do this, shift the weight of your body side-to-side and front-to-back until the weight in both feet feels balanced. If your one or both feet pronate, you'll want to shift the weight from the inner edge of your feet (or foot if only one collapses) to the outer edge until the weight is distributed as evenly as possible. One foot may be different from the other, so double check both feet. Now gently place your toes back down without collapsing the arches. This alone takes time to master. If you have low arches or flat feet, you'll want to repeat this practice throughout your day.

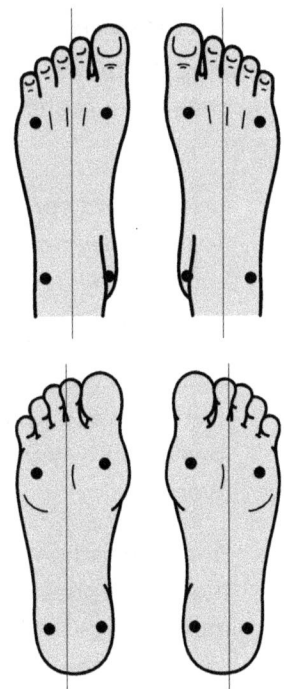

Align the Feet

125

2. Align The Knees

The knees are positively affected by the optimal position of your feet and negatively affected by misalignment of them. The knees—when in balance—typically point towards the middle toes rather than towards the big toes or pinky toes (although there can be exceptions). If your knees roll in towards the big toes, your arches might have collapsed. If so, lift and spread all ten toes which will lift the arches up again. One way to reposition the knees is to firmly set the feet, bend the knees, turn them towards the middle toes, and re-straighten the legs. Make sure not to lock your knees, because that can also negatively impact your lower back.

3. Align the Pelvis

Aligning the pelvis is a three-part process. To move the biggest bones of the body (femurs and ilium), you've got to tone your leg muscles. So, here goes . . . .

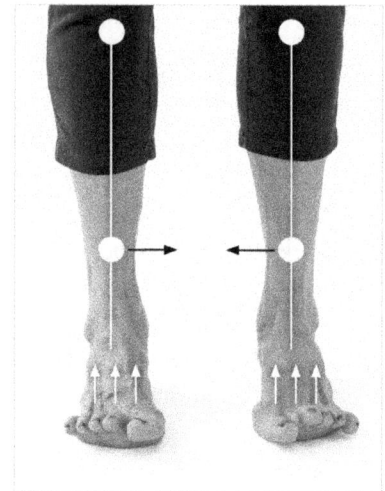

Align Knees

1.   First, lift and spread your toes, while hugging your feet and shins isometrically towards one another—without moving your feet at all. You'll feel the outer calf and inner thigh muscles get stronger. Keep hugging your feet and shins as you proceed.

2.   Second, shift the top of your thigh bones back deeper into the hip sockets by moving the front of the groin backwards making the V-shaped 'hollow' even deeper. This action will move the sitting bones back and apart and tip the whole pelvis a little forward. Tipping the pelvis forward deepens the curve in the lower back (which will feel good if your "cocktail pose" is to flatten your lower back, or worse if you tend to overarch).

3.   Finally, lengthen the tailbone down and forward—just a little—towards the pubic bone, without pushing the thigh bones or pubic bone forward or tucking the sitting bones under! As you drop the tailbone, you must engage the lower abdominals (between the pubic bone and navel). That deep muscular action starts to support the lower back. Then press down through the legs to ground the lower body.

This is a subtle movement that may be mastered over time because it takes sensitivity to balance these movements. How do you know when your pelvis is in balance? The pubic bone, navel, right ASIS, and left ASIS will all be level with one another. And the ASIS and sacroiliac joints (SI joints) will also be level on the horizontal plain. Looking in a mirror, you can place one finger on the front hip bone and another on the SI joint. Are they level? Or is one higher than the other? If the front is higher, move your thigh bones and sit bones back further (over the knees and ankles) until the two spots are level. If the back (SI) is higher than the front, drop your tailbone down a little until they are level.

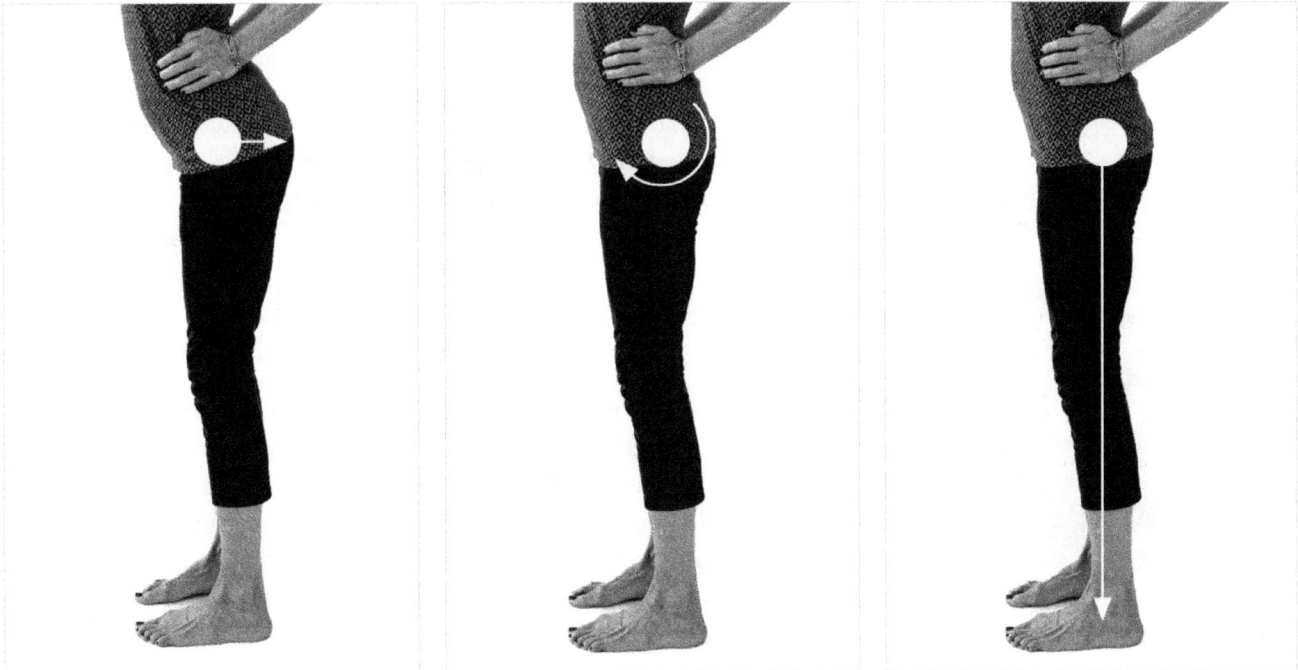

Thighs Back and Tailbone Down

Standing: Align the Upper Body (Grow)

Now that you know how to align the lower body, it's time to look at the upper body—the spine, neck, head, shoulders, arms and hands. When the body is optimally aligned, there is ease and freedom of movement. The vertebrae and joints are properly stacked, reducing gravitational pressure on the spine. Since the body has lots of moving parts, I'd suggest you practice and become familiar with each section—and then put them all together. You'll know you're properly aligning because your body will feel stronger, your breath will become deeper and you'll feel more alive.

Let's identify important markers so you can begin to realign properly:

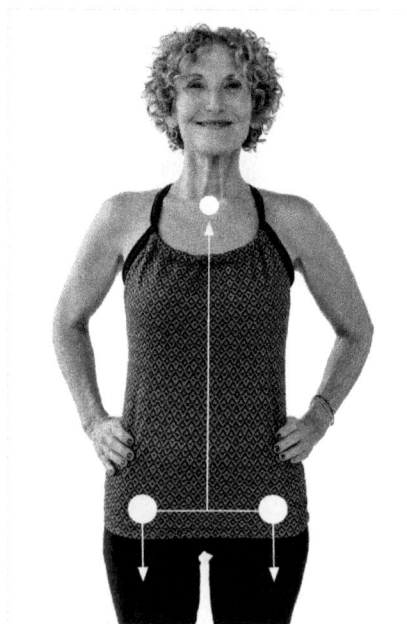

Align the Spine

1. The Spine

In chapter seven, I described the four natural curves of the spine—sacral, lumbar, thoracic, cervical—in detail. It's important to know that your bone structure dictates how deep or shallow your curves are. Slender-boned people tend to have more shallow curves and big-boned folks tend to have deeper curves. But every one's body has the same basic curves. If imbalanced posture causes any curve to become exaggerated or reversed, you might experience back pain. Correcting misalignment should relieve the same pain that a misalignment causes. Remember, the sacral and thoracic areas of the spine curve out (kyphotic) while the lumbar and cervical areas curve in (lordotic).

In order for the vertebrae to shift into their natural position, it's imperative to make enough room for them to do so. Once the legs and pelvis are aligned (feet parallel, thighs back, and tailbone down), you can draw the spine up out of the pelvis during inhalation. Rooting the tailbone anchors the base of the spine, allowing you to extend the spine upward through the head. This is the same self-traction technique from chapter ten. Extending the spine evenly on all sides activates the psoas, abdominal muscles, and back muscles, preserving the alignment of the lower back.

The easiest way to practice this is to align the lower body while resting your hands on your hips (fingers facing forward, thumbs facing back). Once you've moved the sit bones back, dropped the tailbone down, and toned the lower abs, it's time to "ground and grow." Bend your knees slightly, take a deep breath in, and as you exhale, straighten both legs. As you inhale, press your hands down on your hips and lengthen your spine from the tailbone up to the top of your head. Hold this position for several breaths to make an imprint in your body and mind.

2. The Shoulder Girdle

It's best to align the shoulder girdle upon inhalation. As you breathe in and lengthen your spine (with hands on hips), draw the upper arm bones (humerus) straight up into the shoulder sockets until they are in line with the base of your neck. Then, externally rotate the upper arms by drawing both elbows back until you feel both shoulder blades comfortably snug in the back of your ribcage. Keep the shoulder blades in place and breathe deeply, careful not to pinch the shoulder blades onto the spine—there needs to be space so the vertebrae and lungs can move. And make sure to keep the upper abdominals strong, otherwise the back ribs will push the front ribs forward, hardening the spinal muscles. Aligning the shoulder girdle corrects slouchy shoulder and text neck syndromes, which is so very common in modern culture as people look down at books, tablets, pads, laptops, and phones. Looking down all the time can exacerbate chronic back pain and make you feel depressed.

3. The Arms & Hands

Once your shoulder blades rest snuggly on the back ribs, release your hands and rest them by the sides of your body without letting go of this new shoulder alignment or dropping the arms out of the shoulder

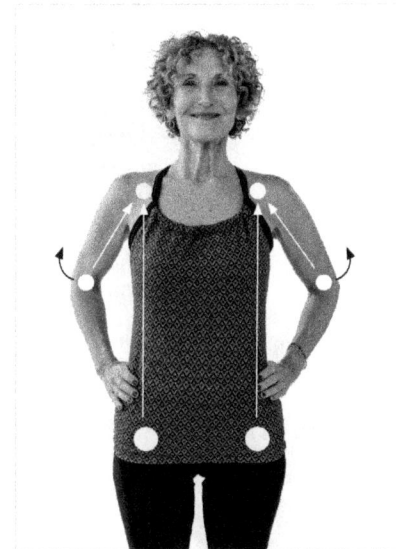

Align the Arms and Hands

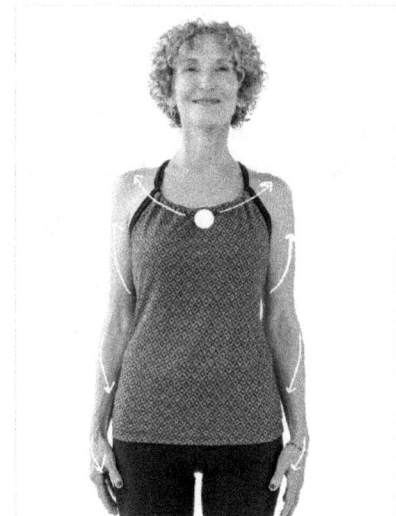

Align the Neck and Head

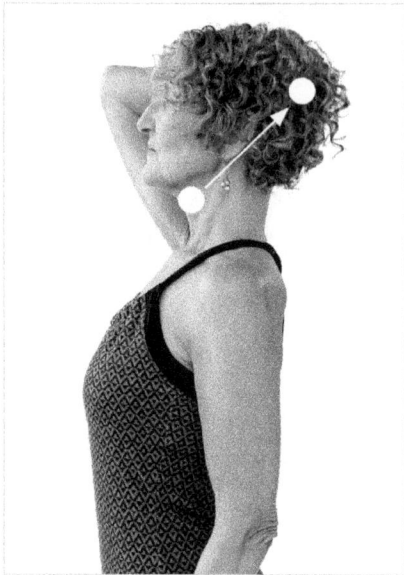

Align the Neck and Head

sockets. Externally rotating the upper arms will turn the forearms and palms away from the legs. So, keeping the upper arms and shoulder blades steady, internally rotate the forearms from the elbow to the wrist, turning the palms to face the thighs. These opposite actions are similar to wringing out a wet cloth—the upper arms turn out and the forearms turn in to properly align the shoulder girdle.

4. The Head

In a neutral position, the head floats freely on top of the spine, in line with the spinal axis. The eyes look forward out to the horizon, not down to the ground or up to the sky. Once you've lengthened your spine and adjusted the shoulder girdle, slide your head slightly back and up so the ears float directly above the shoulders, hips, tailbone, knees, and feet. Make sure to keep your gaze steady on the horizon as you do this. Tucking the chin flattens the curve of the neck, lifting the chin exaggerates the curve and both movements compress the discs of the neck. If you habitually lift your chin, slide your head straight back and lift the occiput slightly up, so your chin lowers down to neutral and the eyes return to the horizon. If you habitually tuck your chin and flatten your neck, lift your forehead slightly up and bring the eyes to the horizon, and slide your head straight back. Either way, when the head moves back into proper alignment with the rest of the spine, you'll feel your abdominal muscles tone, your toes stretch forward (to keep you from falling backwards), and your spine extend up against gravity.

Don't you feel taller? Stronger? Can you observe a deeper breath and a little less pain?

Write down your observations:

_____

_____

_____

_____

OPTIMAL ALIGNMENT IN EVERYDAY POSTURE

Now it's time to take the basic biomechanical alignment and apply it to everyday positions like standing, sitting, walking, bending, twisting, lifting and reclining. As these are the positions you use most of the time, this is where you can really begin to help yourself get out of pain and back on track! Quickly, you'll see how the same blueprint applies in every position and you'll be on your way to creating a healthy, happy back. I'll teach you pain-free walking, supported standing, savvy sitting, better bending, lightly lifting, terrific twisting, and luxurious laying down— all using the same basic biomechanical principles of alignment. I'll also discuss the ergonomics of sitting, because that's one major cause of chronic back pain in today's overly sedentary culture.

It's also important to recognize if your back pain is from underuse (too much sitting or standing), overuse (too much movement), or misuse (incorrect posture whether moving or stationary). When you do, you'll have useful information to select the best practices to balance your whole body.

Pain-free Standing: (Stand Tall)

Practice aligning your standing position in front of a full-length mirror and watch how your "cocktail pose" transforms into a strong and beautiful standing pose.

1. **Stand with your feet and legs hip-distance apart and parallel.** Remember, hip-distance is marked by the hip sockets or by the bones on the front of the pelvis—not by the flesh of your outer hips! It's where the ball of thigh (femur) bone fits into the hip socket (acetabulum). You can also locate this by placing your fingertips on the front hip bones that stick forward. Separate your feet so the center of each ankle and knee are positioned directly below the center of each hip socket. Adjust your feet so that the second toes of each foot are parallel to one another and in line with the center of each ankle. Adjust the center of each heel so it is parallel to the other heel and in line with the center of the ankle. (Look over one shoulder and down to the heels to check your precision.) Now, take a deep breath in and out. Keep breathing!

2. **Lift and spread all ten toes (even inside your shoes).** This will engage the inner (medial) and outer (lateral) arches of both feet. Keep the arches lifted, as you lightly press all ten toes back down into the floor to engage the plantar muscles on the bottom of your feet and lift the metatarsal arches. If the arches drop when you replace your toes, you'll want to practice with all ten toes lifted.

3. **With toes spread and rooted and arches lifted, pull your feet and shins towards one another without moving them (isometric).** This action will tone the muscles of your inner thighs (adductors).

4. **Slightly bend your knees so you don't lock them, and keep them unlocked as you continue.**

5. **While hugging feet and shins, slide the inner thighs (groins) back so the pelvis tips forward and the sit bones move backwards and apart.** This movement should line up the hip sockets directly over the ankles and create a curve in your lower back.

6. **Keeping that action steady, slide your tailbone down and forward toward the pubic bone—just a little—not enough to push the thigh bones (now nicely tucked deep into the hip sockets) or the pubic bone forward.** When done correctly, you'll feel the lower abdominal muscles tone and the naval draw back inwards to the spine, toning the middle abdominals. Now take another deep breath in and out. As you exhale, look down at your feet and squeeze your upper abdominals, drawing the lowest front ribs closer together. On the next inhale, lift your head back to the horizon. Now the entire 6-pack abdominals are toned. That's core strength—without doing a hundred crunches.

7. **Next ground (press) down through the pelvis and legs into the earth and straighten your legs without locking your knees.**

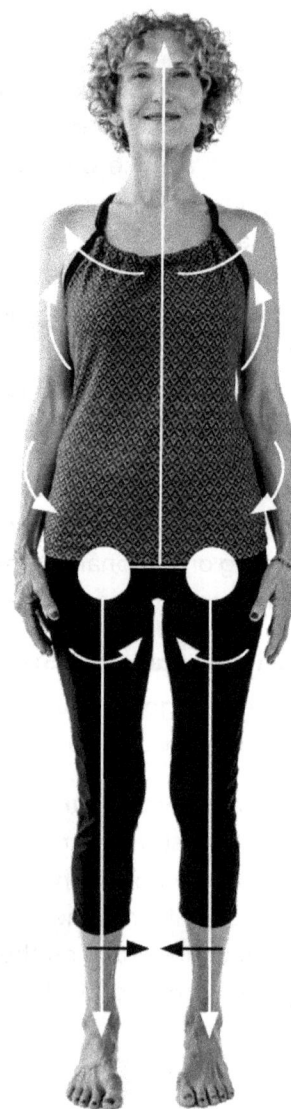

Pain-Free Posture

8. **Simultaneously, grow (lengthen) your spine from the tip of the tailbone to the top of your head, lifting your sternum and ribcage up away from the hips.** Breathe deeply, filling the lungs and ribcage up evenly on all sides. Keep your breastbone (sternum) lifted.

9. **With the next inhalation, gently lift your upper arm bones (humerus) into their shoulder sockets, until the tops of both shoulders line up with the base of your neck.** Then gently move the arm bones back, engaging the upper back muscles (rhomboids) between the shoulder blades. (*Note:* This action is best done by externally rotating the upper arm bones as you lift the chest, arms and shoulders). Here, the biceps move forward and away from the chest, engaging the upper back muscles. As you exhale, make sure that you don't pull the tops of the arm bones down out of the shoulder sockets—or you'll go back to the slouchy posture you had before.

10. **Finally, lift your head and look straight forward—eyes to the horizon, and taking another deep breath in and out, slide the base of the skull back and slightly up.** When done correctly, the ears will move back and up slightly, and the chin will soften down a little. Here, your head will be in a neutral (pain-free) position sitting proudly atop your spine.

Well done! You've just successfully aligned your body in accordance with biomechanical principles, and now your shoulder, hip, knee, and ankle joints are all properly stacked. The force of gravity isn't stuck in the vertebrae of your spine because you're in a perfect plumb line. The muscles of your feet, calves, quadriceps, abdominals, and upper back are evenly toned. Don't you feel stronger and taller? Congratulations—because you just learned how to build a strong, steady, structurally aligned standing pose from the feet to the head—the optimal back care blueprint.

QUICK TIPS FOR STANDING TALL

1. Stand with feet hip distance apart and parallel.

2. Lift and spread all ten toes.

3. Hug feet and shins isometrically to engage inner thigh muscles.

4. Move inner thighs (groins) and sit bones back.

5. Scoop the tailbone down towards the pubic bone to tone the lower abs. Draw the navel back to tone the middle abs. Draw the lower front ribs down and in to tone the upper abs.

6. Ground legs down into earth and lengthen spine from tailbone to head.

7. Move head back and up slightly until the ears are directly over the shoulders, hips, knees and ankles. Make sure the chin is a bit lower than the base of the skull and your gaze looks out to the horizon.

Pain-Free Walking: (Walking Tall)

Walking is a great way to release tension, especially when back pain arises from lack of movement, too much sitting, or underuse. Once you've got the hang of standing tall, you'll want to walk with the same proper alignment as you move through your day. This can be tricky because it's likely there's a pattern of misalignment when you walk—your personal "walking cocktail pose." This misalignment could have the same pattern as your "standing cocktail pose" or a different one.

First, follow the instructions for standing tall to establish optimal alignment. (Demonstration sequence on following page.)

1. **Maintain an aligned upright posture as you walk.**

2. **Keep your head level and your gaze on the horizon.**

3. **Keep your feet pointing straight ahead, not turned out (duck-toe) nor turned in (pigeon-toe).**

4. **Feel the ground beneath your feet as you walk, sensing any shifts on the floor or sidewalk with your feet.** This way you'll feel steadier overall.

5. **When you walk, use all the muscles of your feet.** Strike the floor with the heel of the front foot and roll onto the outer edge of the foot to the little toe mound, and push off the back foot with the big toe mound.

6. **Don't stomp around flat-footed because that can agitate the lower back.**

Make sure to look ahead, eyes to the horizon, not down to the floor or ground, so you don't lose that lovely alignment. Remember, dropping your head down and forward pulls your whole spine out of alignment. It also disengages the upper abdominals which are often the weakest muscles in the body. Avoid walking while looking down at your cell phone, as this over stretches the neck and upper back muscles. If you are walking outdoors on uneven terrain, look down with your eyes rather than your head unless absolutely necessary. Track the feet and knees in line with the hip sockets as you walk. Allow your hips to sway side to side. Keep your head over your shoulders and your shoulders over the hips. These tips will ensure that your abdominals and upper back muscles stay engaged and improve balance. Stay firm in the abdominals as you walk (or run)—especially those upper abdominals! Breathe deeply and use the expansion of each inhalation to lift your chest up and open, as this will help to elongate your spine and decompress the vertebrae.

Make sure to lift the upper arm bones (humerus) into the shoulder sockets. Externally rotate the upper arm bones away from the chest just enough to draw both shoulder blades onto the ribcage, a little closer to the spine—this keeps you from slouching. Now, rotate the forearms so the palms of your hands face in towards your hips. Allow your arms to swing gently without letting them hang off the shoulder sockets. Hanging arms and slouchy posture stresses the neck muscles and spinal discs.

Note: If your pattern when standing up straight is to push the whole rib cage forward, military-style, you may have the same pattern when walking.

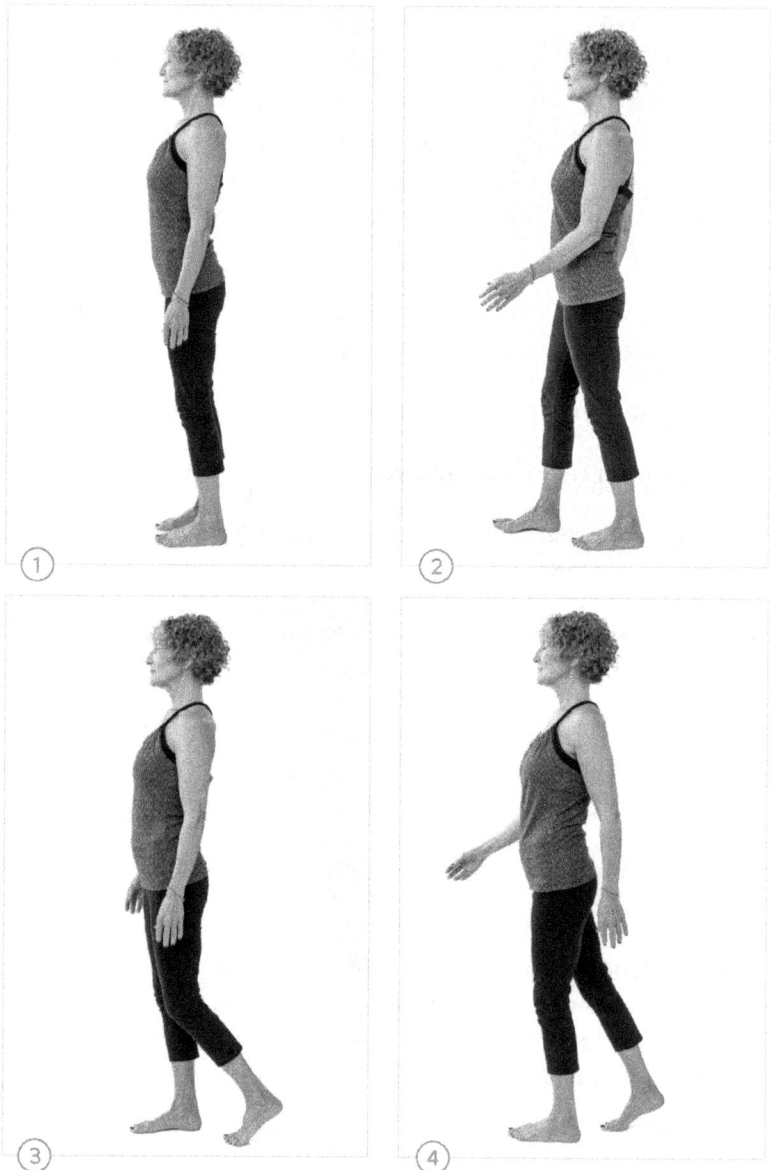

Pain-Free Walking

Pushing the chest forward hardens the lower and mid-back muscles and weakens the abdominals. It also increases back pain. It's best to keep your abdominal muscles strong and back muscles relaxed as you walk. To correct military posture when walking, practice this:

Maintain an optimal standing position and look down at your toes. As you exhale, draw the front lower ribs in towards one another and down towards the navel by toning the upper abdominals. Maintain strong upper abdominals as you lift your gaze back up to the horizon. Readjust the shoulder blades onto the back ribs and slide your head back without lifting the chin. Now, stand and walk tall. The practice will teach you to equally engage both the abdominal and back muscles.

As you walk, it may feel as though you are leaning back a bit more than you are accustomed. With your head stacked over your shoulders, hips, knees, and ankles you'll eventually discover a new more upright gate—great alignment on the go!

QUICK TIPS FOR WALKING TALL

1. Walk with your gaze to the horizon, not to the ground.

2. Keep your abdominal muscles strong and back muscles relaxed.

3. Lift your head up towards the sky to create more space in between the vertebrae.

4. Gently self-traction your spine as you go about your day.

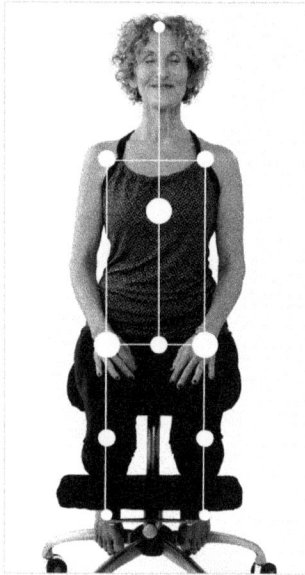

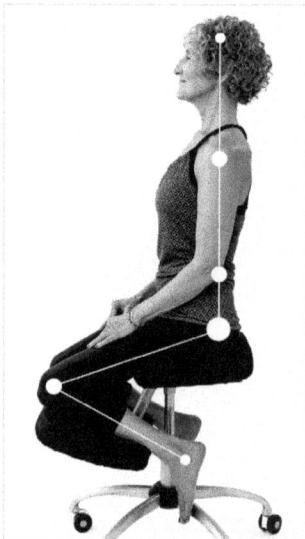

Pain-Free Sitting (Savvy Sitting)

Since most people who sit all day complain about lower back pain, it's important to get savvy with sitting. Sitting uses most of the same alignment cues as standing tall posture. The foundation is both the sitting bones and the feet.

The Ergonomic Seat

The way you adapt your surroundings to your particular physical proportions is called ergonomics. The type of chair you sit on all day is as important as the way you sit on it. But not all chairs or seats are created equally. Basically, any type of seat where the back edge of the seat is lower than the front edge is bad for your back!! Bucket car seats are a no-no. Adirondack chairs, though quaint, are very hard on the buttocks and back. And once you get in, you can barely get out. Soft couches are downright harmful for your back because they make your spine slouch more. Any cushion that's not firm enough to hold your weight steady without letting you sink down into it can be a cause of chronic back pain. And while generally a firmer cushion is better for your back than a soft squishy cushion, some seats are just too darn hard for bony people to go without a little cushioning. The ideal is to find the right seat and the right amount of cushioning to adequately support your spine.

Here's what you must know about sitting:

For savvy sitting without pain, your hips sockets must be slightly higher than your knee joints. A slightly forward-tipping pelvis allows for a natural curve of your lower back. If you have a seat that tips your pelvis backward and flattens your lower back (like a bucket seat), put a firm cushion underneath your sit bones to prop your hips up above your knees. You can do this at your desk, in your car, at the dining room table—make sure ALL of your seats are working for you, not against you.

The height of the chair should match the length of your shins so your feet can rest comfortably flat on the floor—not hanging in the air—which can strain the hips and lower back. Adjustable chairs are great for this reason because you can change their height to match your body size. Basically, you want to sit the same way you stand, with a few modifications. When you sit, you have two choices: slide your pelvis all the way to the back of the seat or sit on the front edge of the seat. I prefer the second choice because you won't slouch into the backrest of the chair. Either way, place your feet flat on the floor (or on a cushion, if the seat is taller than your shins are long).

To find the optimal position of the pelvis: place your feet, shins, and thighs parallel and hip-distance apart. Then, rock your sitting bones forward and backward to find the center point. This is the place where your spine lengthens up, supporting the weight of your head, and allowing all four spinal curves to stack properly. Be aware that tipping the pelvis too far backwards flattens the lower back and rounds your spine and shoulders, while rocking the sit bones too far forward hardens the back muscles and overarches your lower back.

Once you feel balanced in the sitting bones, draw your tailbone down towards the chair seat and tone up through your lower and middle abdominal muscles. (*Tip:* To engage the upper abs gaze down at your lap, exhale and draw the front ribs down towards the hips. Then, keep the upper abs toned as you lift your head and shoulders back up to a neutral position.)

Do not allow your knees to splay apart and do not slouch into the back of the chair. Both misalignments shift the weight from the sitting bones (where they are meant to be) onto the sacrum, over-rounding the lower back. This common position flattens the lower back, creates undue tension and pain in the sacroiliac joints (SI), and risks injury or reinjury. Ouch! Please stop slouching when you sit.

Now, take a deep breath in and fill up your ribcage. Move your shoulders up and back to engage upper back muscles. Then lift your gaze and move your head/ears back over your shoulder and your shoulders back over your hips. When done correctly, you'll have equal strength in the upper back and belly muscles. Your neck won't get sore and neither will your upper back. And you'll be on your way to correcting slouchy shoulder syndrome, at least while you sit.

Maintain this optimal posture while breathing fully.

66 ————

You want to sit the way you stand.

> **Your body is designed to bend from the hip sockets.**

Pain-Free Bending (Better Bending)

Bending is an everyday movement that moves the spine into a forward bend, flattening the lumbar spine and overstretching the mid-back and neck muscles. Much of daily life is spent in a constant forward bend, so it's important to train yourself to bend properly, reducing overuse and misuse that increases the risk of chronic reinjury. Your body is designed to bend from the hip sockets, but the majority of people bend from the waist and spine instead. No wonder millions of people are in so much pain. The hip sockets are designed to be the main pivot point between the upper and lower body. Using your hips properly will take the load of gravity out of your lower back and reduce chronic pain in the spine.

In order to bend properly, there are two options:

Bending with a neutral spine and straight legs or bending with a neutral spine and bent knees. If you are reaching for something that is lightweight and easy to reach, use the first method—neutral spine with straight legs. Some people call this 'flat

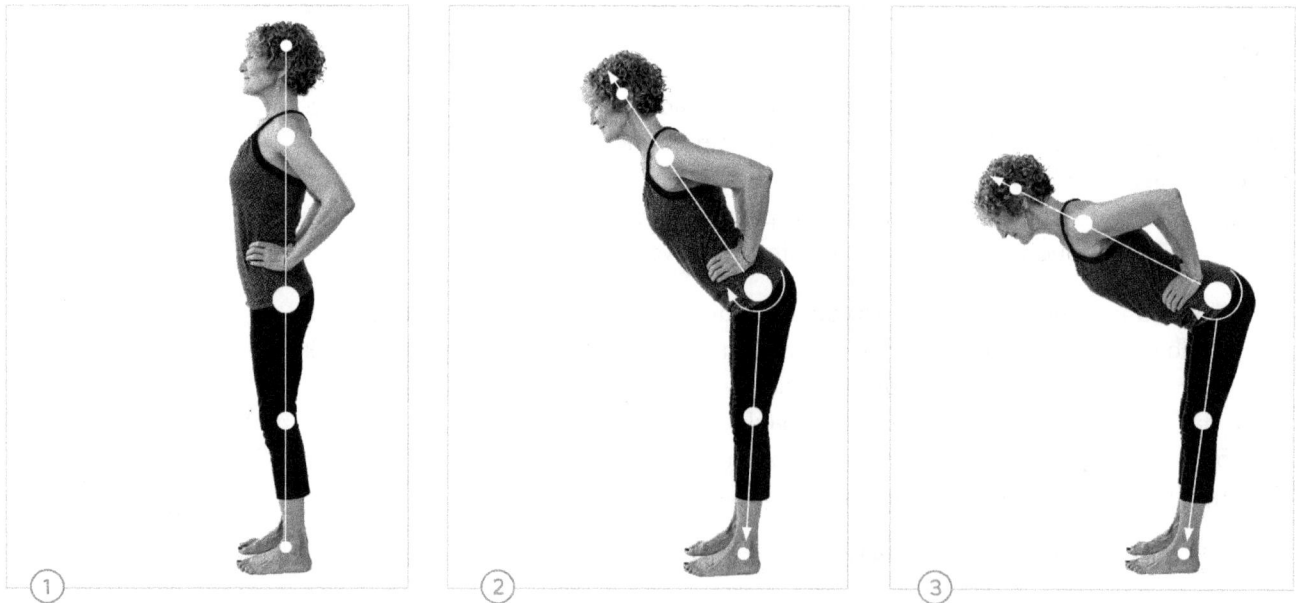

back', which is a misnomer because you want to preserve the natural curve of your lower back, not flatten it. If you're reaching for something heavy, use the second position with bent knees.

Straight Leg

Start in the 'standing tall' stance from page 131: Taking a deep breath in, hug the feet and shins towards one another. As you exhale, fold forward from the hip sockets pushing the sit bones back as far as you can, and tuck the tailbone down and under to tone the abdominals in and up. Try to maintain the natural curve of the spine and strong muscles in the legs and abs.

When you're ready to stand back up, take another deep breath in, and on the exhale push down through your legs, pivot on the hip sockets to lift the whole upper body—spine, shoulders, arms and head—together as one unit.

Tip: Instead of standing with your feet parallel, you can step one foot forward and the other foot behind, so your stance is 2–3 feet long. This will increase the overall stability of your whole body. Before you bend forward, press your back leg down through the heel, grounding into the floor. Shift the weight from the front

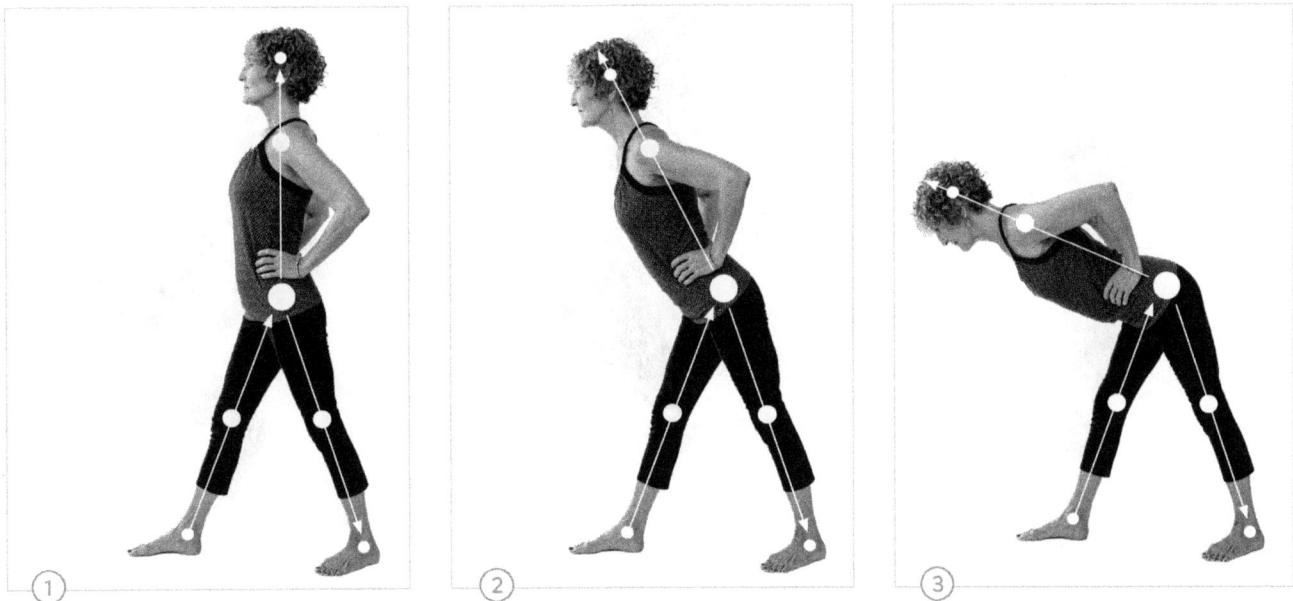

leg to the back leg until they're equally weighted. This will ease the gravitational pressure on your spine.

If the neutral spine/straight leg method puts too much pressure into your lower back, try the following bent knee method instead.

Bent Knee

Stand tall, take a big breath in, hugging the feet and knees towards one another. As you exhale, bend both knees forward and push both sit bones back as far as you can (as if you were about to sit down on a chair). Make sure your lower back arches in, not out! Now, tuck your tailbone, strengthen the abdominals, and squat as deeply as you comfortably can. When you're ready to come up, take another deep breath in, and as you exhale, press your legs and feet down into the floor and stand up straight and tall, lifting the object safely.

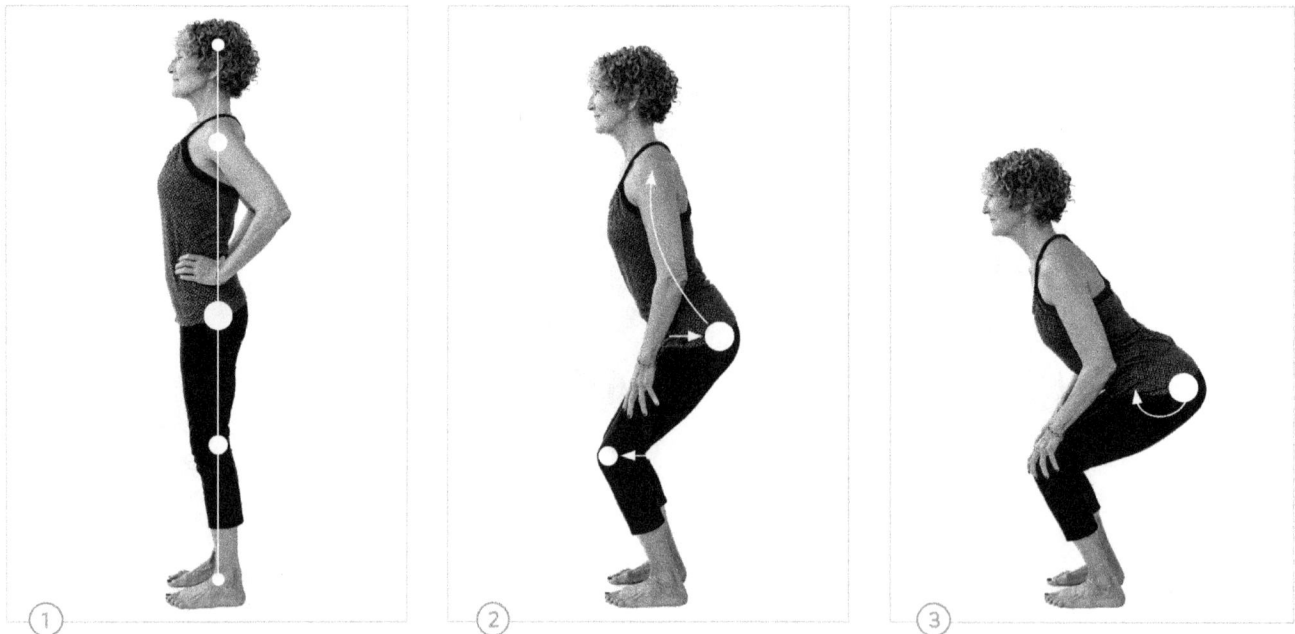

Pain-Free Lifting (Lightly Lifting)

Again, you can choose to lift with straight legs or bent knees. If you're lifting something that's not too heavy or too far away, you can use the first method—straight legs with a neutral spine. If you are lifting something heavy, use the bent knee position.

Straight Legs

This is ideal when lifting lightweight objects. Start with your "standing tall" stance, take a big breath in, and as you exhale, fold forward from the hip sockets as far as you can while maintaining the natural curve of your spine, and reach out with your arms and grab whatever you're after. Pull it close to your chest, engaging the back and arm muscles. You'll want to use your arm strength as much as your back and leg strength.

Tip: instead of standing with your feet parallel, step one foot forward and the other foot back, so your stance is about 2–3 feet long. A longer stance will increase your overall stability. Before you bend forward, press from your hips down through your back leg and foot, rooting them into the floor. That action will shift some weight away from your front leg and spine, easing the pressure on them both.

Bent Knees

If that method puts too much pressure in your lower back, or you're lifting something heavy, try the bent knee method instead. (Guide photos on following page.)

Stand in your "standing tall" stance, and take a big breath in. As you exhale, bend both knees forward and push both sit bones back as far as possible (as if you were about to sit down into a chair) so your lower back arches! Then scoop your tailbone down and under to strengthen your abdominal muscles. Next, bend as deeply as you can. Then, reach out with your arms and pull whatever you're lifting close into your body. Move your shoulders back to re-engage your upper back muscles!

Take another breath in, and as you exhale, press down through your legs and feet into the floor (diving board) and stand back up straight and tall.

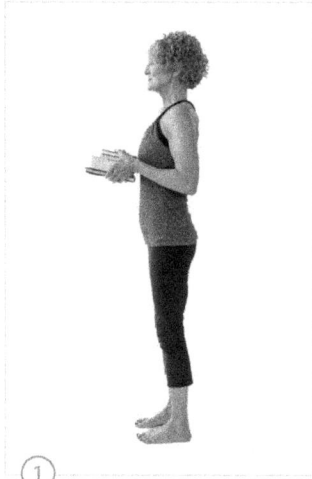

①

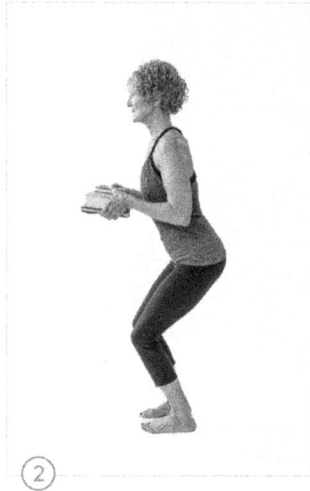

②

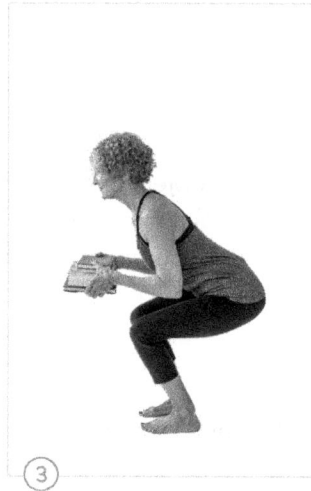

③

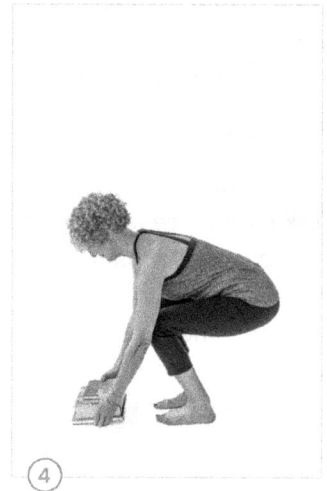

④

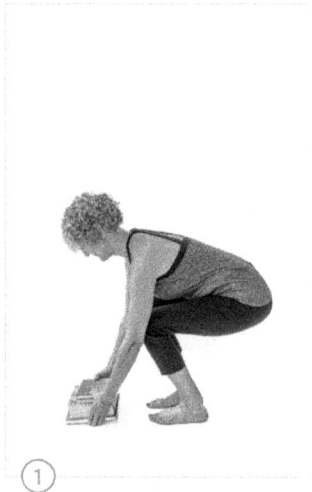

①

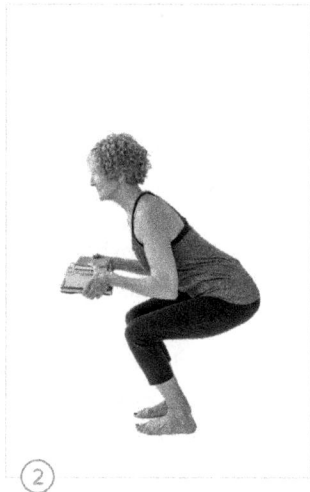

②

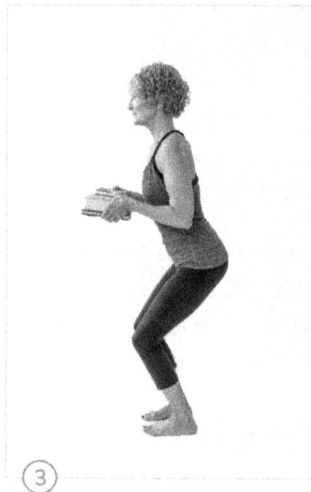

③

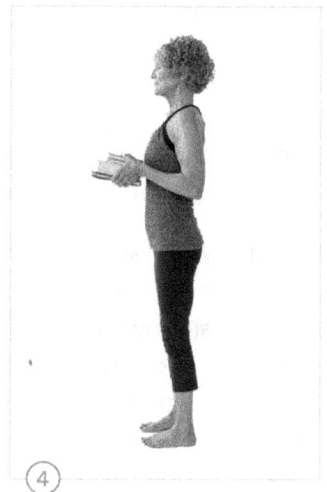

④

Pain-Free Twisting (Terrific Twisting)

Pain-free twisting combines elements of both bending and lifting or reaching, so it's important to move slowly so you can discover how you might be causing back pain! There are three common tendencies in unmindful twisting: the first is to move too quickly, jerking the upper body away from the lower body. The next pattern is to move the most mobile body parts first—the arms, neck, and head—which can strain the less mobile parts of your body—the middle, lower back, and sacrum. The third common tendency is to twist in an unorganized manner, thus creating more misalignment instead of ensuring optimal alignment as you twist.

To prevent straining or tweaking your back when twisting, here are a few suggestions:

If you're standing upright and need to reach for something to your right or left side, take a big breath in, hugging your feet and shins towards one another, and strengthening the legs. Breathe out and root down through your legs as you lift up through your spine. Tone your abdominal muscles. Keep your pelvis facing in the same direction as your feet to protect the sacrum. If you absolutely must turn your hips, it's better to turn your feet and legs in the direction of the twist to reduce the load on your spine. Upon exhaling, keep the length of your spine and twist your upper body in order of lower back, lower ribs, middle ribs, shoulders, arms, and head in the direction of choice. Grab whatever item you need on the next inhalation, and draw the object close into your chest on exhalation.

Come out of the twist as follows:

Take another breath in, lengthening your spine, and undo the twist in the opposite order. First, turn your head forward, then your arms and shoulders, then the middle ribs, and finally, untwist the lower ribs until you are back where you started.

For ALL twists—whether you're standing or sitting—it's best to stand tall and move slowly, twisting your body from the lower back up through the chest, neck, head and finally reach out with your arms. Returning to the original position will be just the opposite: retract the arms, re-center the head, and slowly unwind the torso from the twist. Come back to center, standing tall.

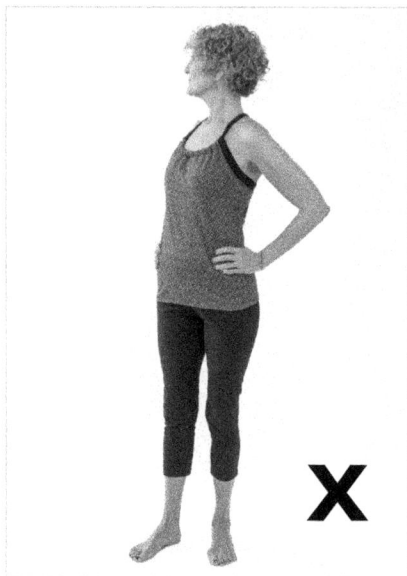

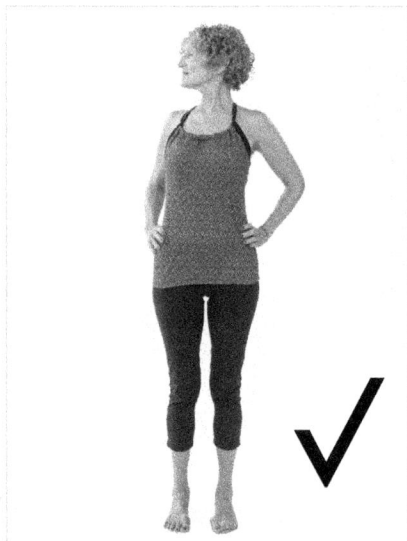

Tip: Bend and twist at the same time.

Use the bent knee method. Bend straight down as far as you can, getting as close to the item you intend to lift as you can. Keep your feet, legs, hips, and torso facing forward. Maintain the natural curve in your lower back, tone the abdominals, keep your shoulders up and back, and engage the upper back muscles (rhomboids). Again, breathe in while hugging your feet, shins, and knees toward one another (even if your knees splayed apart as you bend). Push your sit bones back, and on the exhale, tuck your tailbone under. With your next deep inhalation, lift your spine up away from the hips and keep the abs engaged, and draw your shoulders up and back to engage the upper back muscles.

Now, start the twist from the lower back, lower ribs, middle ribs, shoulders, arms, and finally turn the head. This way you're twisting your spine from bottom to top—from the least mobile part of your spine (sacrum) to the most mobile (head). At this point, you can reach for whatever you're after. It's always best to exhale while moving into a twist because as you twist, you compress the diaphragm, making it harder to breathe in.

Breathing deeply, draw whatever you're lifting close into your body.

Take another inhale, and come out of the twist as you exhale—staying in the bent knee position. Finally, another big breath in, and as you exhale push down through your legs into the floor and stand back upright—all the way back into your Standing Tall stance.

Many people tweak their low back sitting in the front seat of their car as they reach into the back seat to grab something or help their children. This is a very common way to injure your spine because the tendency is to move the arm and head abruptly, forgetting to stabilize the lower body first. It's always best to twist the entire spine—from the lower back/slowest moving part up to the neck and head/fastest moving . . . and always release the twist in the opposite order.

Pain-Free Reclining (Luxurious Laying)

Many people I've met struggle to find comfort when they lay down to rest. So, here's a basic primer for laying down. Consider that laying on your back is essentially the same as standing tall, but you are reclined. Many people sleep with a thick pillow, which creates the same upper body misalignment as the slouchy shoulder or text neck syndrome. Your mattress may be problematic—too hard or too soft, but I'll leave that for you to discern. Whatever surface you lay on, whether a mattress, floor, or carpet, you can follow these instructions to align a belly-up position.

Belly Up (Supine)

Lay down on your back. Place your head and shoulders in line with your hips. Walk your feet 6–12 inches wider than your hips and allow your legs to relax. Notice if your lower back is evenly arched, too flat, or too curved. If your lower back is too flat, lift your right buttock up, grab the right sitting bone with your right hand and shift it over to the right. Do the same with the left side. Widening the sitting bones apart will help release the thigh bones and psoas muscle, allowing the lower back to gently lift up. If the lower back curve is too deep, lengthen your tailbone towards your feet, which lengthens the lower back, decreasing the curve. Now, press your elbows down, lift the back of your ribcage up, and tuck the shoulder blades under the ribs. Remember not to pinch them tightly together. Now, check the curve of your neck. Run the fingers of one hand up and down the back of the neck and discern if it is too flat, too curved or gently curved. Lift and lower your chin until the neck curve feels like an even arc. If the curve is too flat, lift the chin. If the curve is too arched, lower your chin. Finally, rest your arms down by your sides several inches away from your hips. Turn the palms face up to keep the shoulders in position.

In this position, your heels, calves, thighs, ribs, shoulder blades, elbows, back of hands, and head will touch the surface of whatever you're lying on. The back of your ankles, knees, lower back, and neck should not. It is okay to place a little support under these lifted areas (like a rolled towel), but only to fill in the space between your back and the surface—not to push your body into greater misalignment. Once you are comfortable, close your eyes and breathe deeply, allowing stress and pain to release with each exhalation. Maybe now you'll fall asleep.

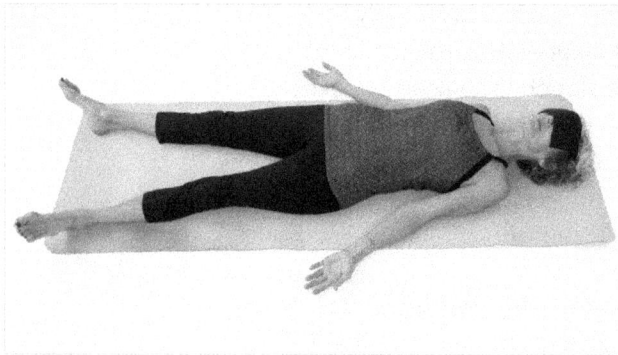

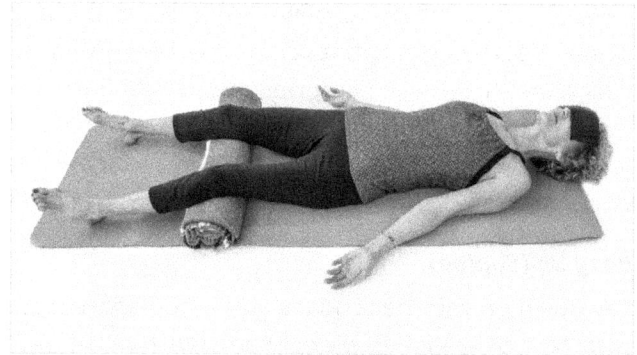

Tip: If laying on your back causes discomfort in your lower back, place a rolled blanket under the back of your knees.

Belly Down (Prone)

If you are someone who is completely uncomfortable laying on your back, here's a different pain-relieving position for you. This alternative position, laying on your belly, can relieve tightness, tension and pain in the lower back.

To do this in a supportive manner, fold a blanket into a 6-inch wide, 4–6 inch thick, and 3-foot long rectangle. Place the blanket on the floor or mattress and lay, belly down, positioning the leg creases (where the legs join the pelvis) directly on top of the blanket. The knees should rest comfortably on the floor or mattress. If they are up in the air, slide your whole body back until the knees drop down. Then, elongate your spine and lay your belly down. Your lower back will assume a nice downward-arching curve. Fold the arms up by your head or stack your hands and place your forehead on the back of your hands. Rest here, quietly breathing until pain subsides and you feel ready to get up.

It takes commitment, mindfulness and practice to shift old patterns of movement and establish new ones, but it is absolutely possible to do so. Once you discover

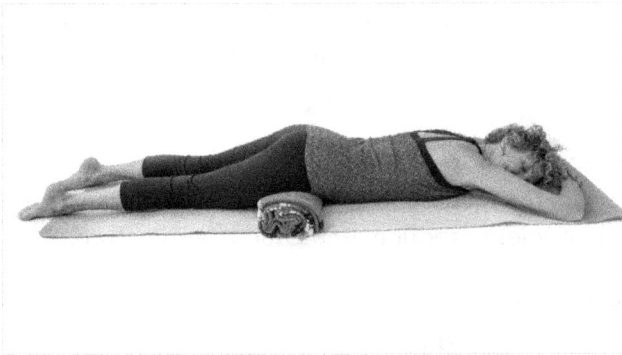

which positions make your back hurt more and which make your back more comfortable, you'll be in command of your own healing journey. Allow each little success to motivate you to stick with this program and sustain the positive changes you've made. Soon, you'll be on your way to healing chronic back pain at home, at work, at play. Well done!!

Correct Your 21st Century Syndrome

Now that I've covered how to adjust your body in everyday postures, I want you to recall the 21st Century syndrome that you discovered in chapter two and the "cocktail pose" you identified in chapter six. Which archetype is your main pattern? Find it (or them) below and use the corresponding tip to help you remember which part of your body needs to be adjusted according to your particular pattern of misalignment. This will simplify the practice.

1) Lumbar Lordosis (Excess Lower Back Curve)

Emphasize the downward movement of the tailbone with the inward and upward tone of the lower and middle abdominal muscles to reduce excess lumbar curvature.

2) Thoracic Kyphosis (Excess Thoracic Curve)

Emphasize the upward lift and external rotation of the upper arm bones with the inward movement of the shoulder blades to stretch pectoral muscles and tone rhomboid muscles.

3) Flat Back (Reversed Lumbar Curve)

Emphasize the backward movement of the thigh bones inside the hip sockets to deepen the lumbar curve.

4) Military Posture (Flat Upper Back/Excess Extension)

Emphasize toning the upper abdominal muscles to draw the lower front ribs downward and inward and expand the back ribs backwards to relax the middle and upper back muscles.

5) Scoliosis (C and S Curves)

C Curve: Tone the muscles on the outer edge of the C curve and stretch the muscles on the inner side of the C curve. If the C curve points to the left side, tone the muscles of the left side of the spine and stretch the muscles of the right side, and vice versa.

S Curve: The S curve is made of two C curves moving in opposite directions (one to the right, other to the left). Use the same strategy as above. For both the lower and upper part of the S curve, tone the muscles of the outer edge of each C curve and stretch the muscles on the inner side of each C curve.

6) Sitter's Disease

Emphasize sitting on the center of the sit bones. Do not slouch onto the back of the sit bones or onto the sacrum. Do not tip too far forward onto the front of the sit bones. Find the midpoint of the sit bones and stay there.

7) Weak Butt

Center your sit bones as recommended in sitter's disease, and press your thigh bones straight down into the chair seat and your feet straight down into the floor. This will tone the buttock muscles and help you extend your spine to resist gravity while you sit.

8) Slouchy Shoulder

Emphasize the upward lift and external rotation of the upper arm bones with the inward and downward movement of the shoulder blades to stretch the pectoral muscles and tone the rhomboid muscles.

9) Text Neck

Emphasize the upward lift and external rotation of the upper arm bones with the inward and downward movement of the shoulder blades to stretch the pectoral muscles and tone the rhomboid muscles. Then, lift the eyes up to the horizon and slide the ears backwards until they're over the shoulder joints.

CONCLUSION

This chapter was jam-packed with specific information to help you realign your whole body and improve your posture so you can move with less pain and more ease. Let's recap the most important principles so you do not feel overwhelmed by all this new information.

1) Ground to Grow

This is the most important biomechanical principle. It teaches you to effectively ground the pressure of gravity down through your legs into the earth and rebound upwards, pushing back against gravity. This technique will unweight your spine, getting the pressure off of the nerves, joints, and discs, to significantly reduce pain fast.

2) Align the Whole Body

Once you've got the hang of "ground to grow", you'll want to practice aligning your body while standing. Then you'll be ready to take your new and improved alignment into walking, sitting, bending, twisting, and reclining (or any other activity you like to do). This will retrain you away from painful old habits and toward new pain-free posture.

3) Take Your Time and Breathe Deeply

Get familiar with these alignment practices. Do not rush, do not force! The more often you adjust your body throughout the day, the less pain you'll experience. In the beginning, you may notice how often you're out of alignment and how often you create pain.

4) Honor Yourself

Never berate yourself for having pain. Your increased awareness is key to ending chronic back pain without pills, shots or surgery. Instead, commend yourself for noticing habitual posture, and adjust accordingly with kindness.

Good alignment is not a "one-time event." It is about improving your relationship with your own body one breath, one position, and one day at a time. Now that we've covered the physical alignment techniques to get you out of pain, let's look at what to do in those difficult moments when back pain flares up and you're unsure of what to do.

CHAPTER 12

TRIAGE FOR CHALLENGING MOMENTS

"For all the happiness mankind can gain:
Is not in pleasure but in rest from pain." — *John Dreyden*

As you continue to become familiar with *The BackCare Blueprint* techniques and practice improving your alignment, remember there will be days, especially in the beginning, when you slip back into old patterns. In those moments, it's important to remember that effecting positive change takes time. The journey to become responsible for your own health and instill effective spinal self-care can present ups and downs. The path you take may wind back and forth between discomfort and ease. This is normal. In moments of great challenge, don't give up! Over time, the trajectory you're on will keep improving as you stick with these practices. Sometimes you might need a "quick fix" to downshift your experience of back pain, and for these moments, I've added a "triage" section to give you additional strategies to reduce back pain on the go. All of these exercises can be done at any time of day and in almost any location, as they do not require a change of clothes or any special equipment. Your own body and the way you align it is the vehicle to get—and keep—yourself out of pain.

TRIAGE FOR PAINFUL STANDING

When you find yourself standing in pain and you cannot get out for a walk, here are three useful exercises to quickly shift the experience of pain. Use them throughout your day as often as you need to make your back feel better.

To begin, stand tall according to the basic postural alignment directions.

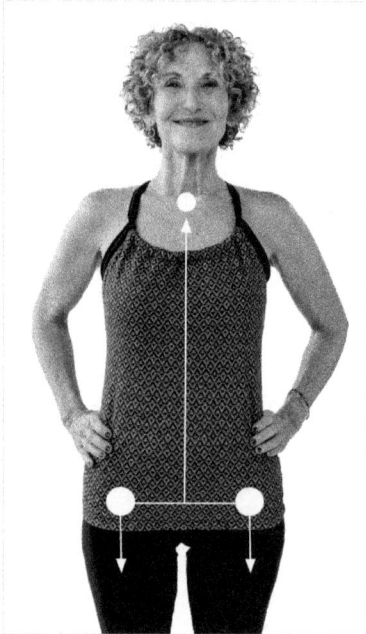

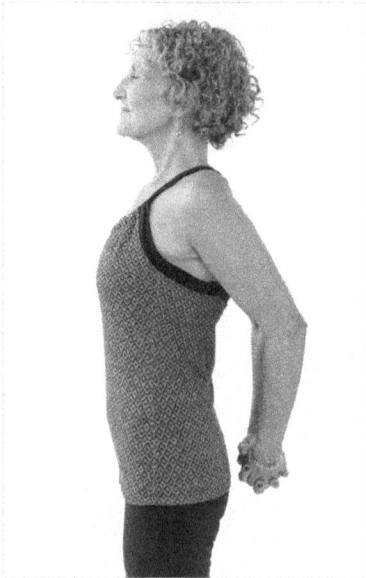

1) General Back Pain

Lift and spread your toes, isometrically hug your feet and shins towards one another, then squeeze your buttock muscles. Hug and release continually for a full minute. Then, hug and hold while breathing deeply for thirty seconds. Release and repeat at least three times, more as needed, if pain persists. Toning the leg and buttock muscles pumps blood through your body, provides support for the spine and enlivens the breath. All may help to reduce pain.

2) Lower Back Pain

Place hands on hips. As you take a deep breath in, press your hands down on the hips and lift the chest, neck and head up to self-traction your spine. Hold this position and breathe for one minute. Release and repeat as often as needed. Self tractioning the spine can give you energy, make you feel more empowered and quickly reduce lower back pain.

3) Upper Back and Neck Pain

Align your whole body and stand tall. Reach your hands behind your back, interlace your fingers resting them on the sacrum. (If you can't reach, place your hands on the back of your hips or hold a strap in both hands). Draw a deep breath in and lift your chest. On the exhalation, straighten your arms, lifting the hands away from your pelvis. Squeeze and release the upper back muscles between your shoulder blades three more times, and squeeze and hold for one minute. Keep breathing! Release and repeat the cycle as many times as you need to relieve upper back pain.

Alternately: Sit on the front edge of your chair seat. Bend your elbows behind you with forearms and hands parallel to the floor. Press both elbows into the back of the chair and push your chest forward then release. Repeat a few times, and then press and hold for thirty seconds. Release and repeat the sequence as many times as you need to relieve tension in the upper back and neck.

TRIAGE FOR PAINFUL SITTING

Sometimes you may be driving in your car or stuck in a meeting where you can't get up and walk around when your back starts to ache. In these situations, whether the muscles suffer from underuse or misuse, it is essential to activate the buttock, leg and back muscles. Here are three simple exercises you can do while sitting to improve sitter's disease, weak butt syndrome, and slouchy shoulder/text neck syndrome. They will tone the buttock, hamstring, quadricep and back muscles. Use them on the go to reduce pain as it arises.

To begin, align your seated position.

1) Sitter's Disease

With legs as wide as your hips, isometrically hug your feet and knees towards one another. Press your thighs straight down into the chair seat and your feet straight down into the floor. Simultaneously, lift your spine up through your head. Hold for 30–60 seconds, breathing deeply. Release and repeat. This will activate the leg muscles, back muscles, and unweight gravity from the lower back.

2) Weak Butt Syndrome

With legs as wide as your hips, isometrically hug your feet and shins towards one another. Press both feet down onto the floor and release. Repeat continually for a full minute. This action will squeeze and release your buttock muscles creating much needed movement for issues of underuse. Now, press the feet, squeeze and hold the buttock muscles, breathing deeply for thirty seconds. Release and repeat. Repeat three times or more, as needed, if pain persists.

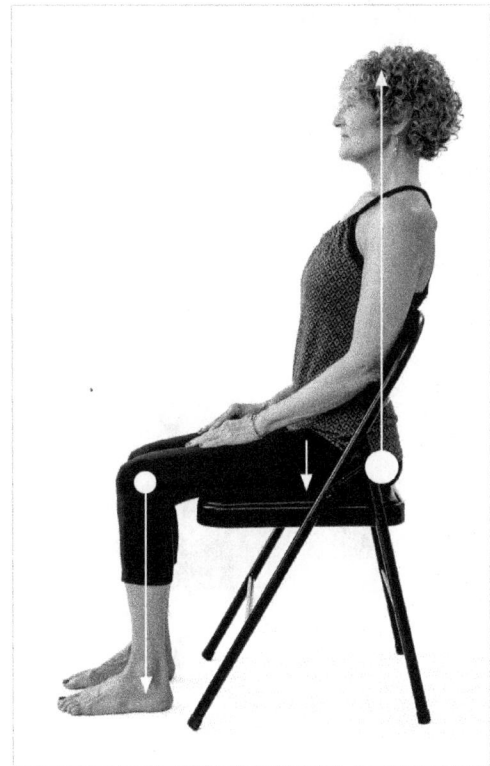

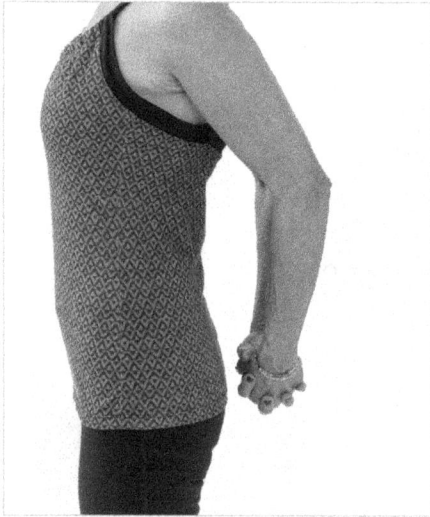

3) Slouchy Shoulder/Text Neck

Turn sideways in your chair (or stand up). Adjust your alignment. Press the sit bones down into the chair and extend your spine up through the head. Clasp both hands behind your back. Start with the elbows bent. Then straighten your arms by moving the hands away from your back to squeeze the upper back and neck muscles. Don't lean forward, keep your head over your hips and only work the upper back muscles. Hold for ten seconds, release, and repeat several times to relieve upper back and neck pain.

4) Leg or Sciatic Pain

With legs as wide as your hips, isometrically hug your feet and shins towards one another. Without moving the feet, isometrically pull both heels back towards the chair legs. This will engage the hamstrings muscles and buttocks to buffer the part of the sciatic nerve that runs down the legs. Breathe continually. Release and repeat several times. Then, pull the feet back and hold for one minute while breathing deeply. Repeat the sequence as often as you need to reduce pain. This exercise can calm the sciatic nerve and reduce sensation.

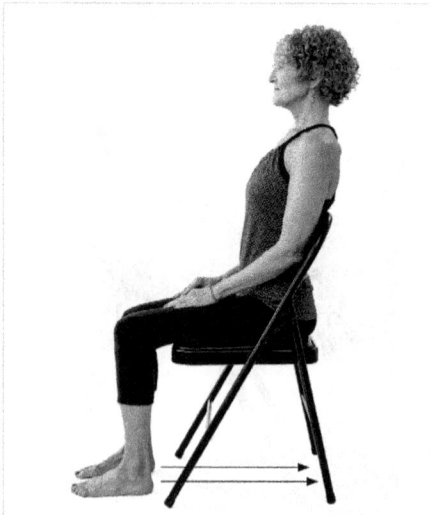

5) General Spinal Tension

Cross the right foot over the left foot (or if possible cross the right knee over the left knee). Hug the feet and knees towards one another and keep that steady. Place the left hand on the outside of the right knee and place the right hand on the right hip. On an inhale, ground down into the sit bones and lengthen the spine up through the top of our head. On the exhale, push down on the right hand while pulling up with the left hand and twist your spine, shoulders, neck, and head—in that order—to the right.

Hold this twist and breathe steadily. If the breath feels restricted, that's normal. On an inhale, extend the spine and move out of the twist and back to center. Repeat a few times on the right side, and repeat on the left side. Notice how the tension in your back has decreased.

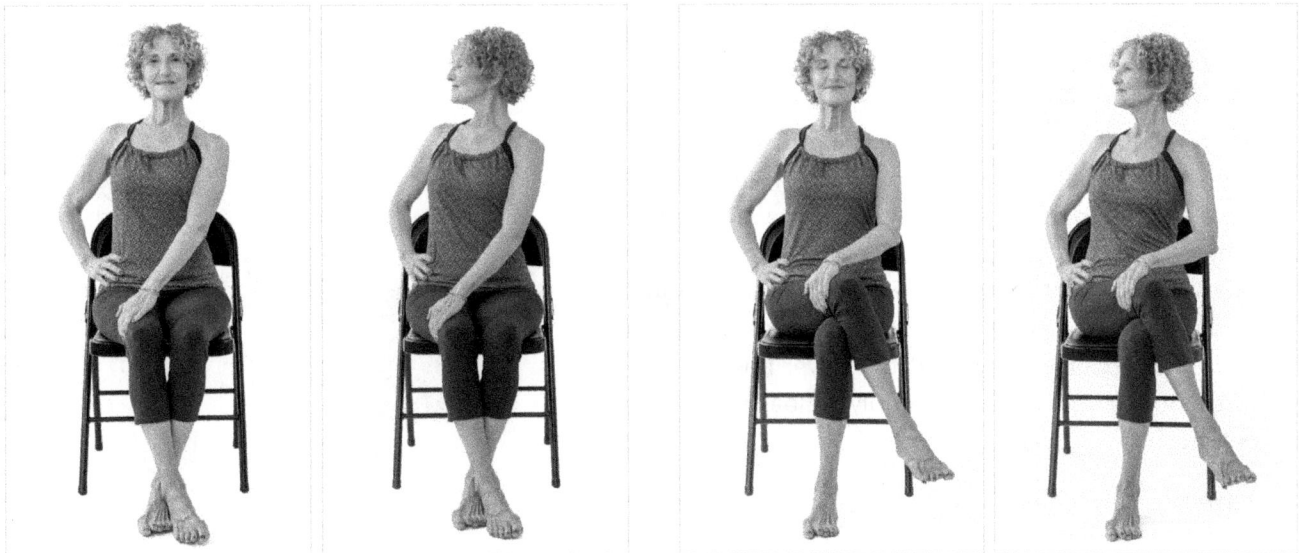

TRIAGE FOR BENDING, LIFTING, TWISTING

This stretch is wonderful for so many reasons and terrific for all kinds of back pain!

You can use it to correct a misalignment from underuse, overuse, or misuse, and to heal pain from repetitive injury because this pose aligns and stretches every part of your body. Practice this when standing or sitting fatigues your body, or when bending, lifting, or twisting strains your back.

1) Standing Dog Pose

Stand an arm length away from any wall. Place both hands on the wall (flat palms or fingertips) a foot or more above the height of your shoulders. Gently hug both wrists and forearms toward one another to tone the biceps. Straighten both arms and bend both knees. Take a deep breath in, and as you exhale, press your arms into the wall and push back evenly through the inner groins and both sit bones. Bend your knees more deeply or walk your feet back away from the wall until you feel a deep stretch from the wrists, down both sides of the lower back, through the groins, and back to the sit bones. Ground the tailbone and tone the abdominals to support the lower back. Hold for thirty seconds as you breathe deeply. Release and repeat a few times.

If the level of lower back pain is high, isometrically squeeze your feet and knees towards one another. Squeeze to match the intensity of the back pain.

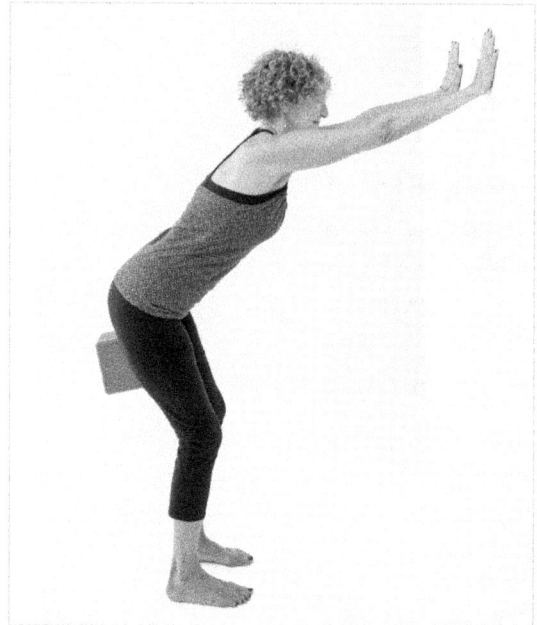

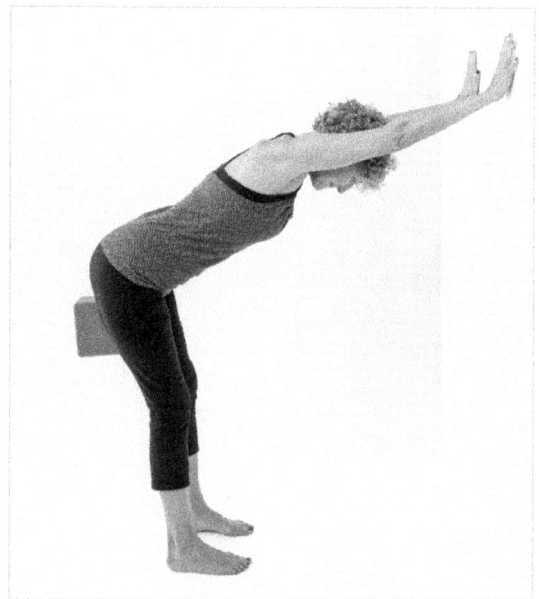

2) Knees to Chest

This is a wonderful pose to do if you've strained your back while bending, lifting, or twisting.

Lay down on your back on a rug, blanket, or mat. Take a few deep breaths. As you exhale, draw the knees towards your chest and hold them with both hands. Relax your face, back, and body, and rest, breathing deeply for a few minutes. Then, press your knees into your hands, straightening your arms, arching your lower back gently. Again, hold and breathe. To release, tone the abdominals and slowly lower your feet to the floor. Then, stretch your legs out long and rest for a minute. To get up, roll to one side, press your hands down into the floor to support your spine as you sit back up.

Tip: You can also practice knees to chest holding one leg at a time. If you notice that one position (drawing close or pressing away) feels better than the other, use that one regularly.

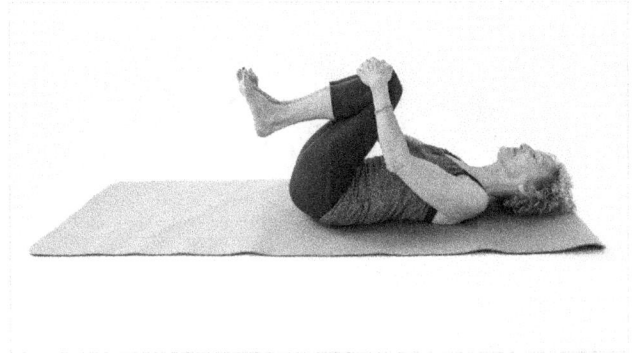

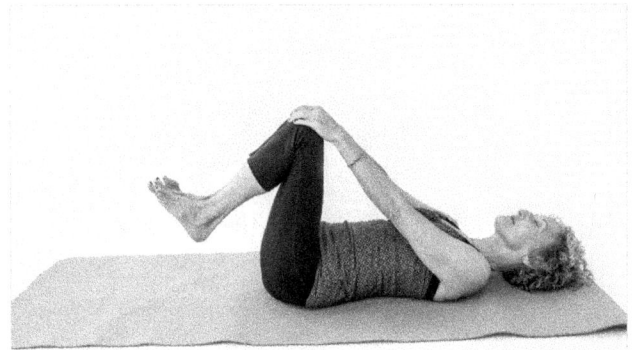

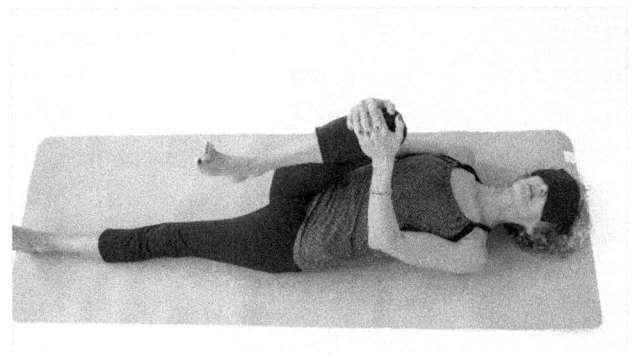

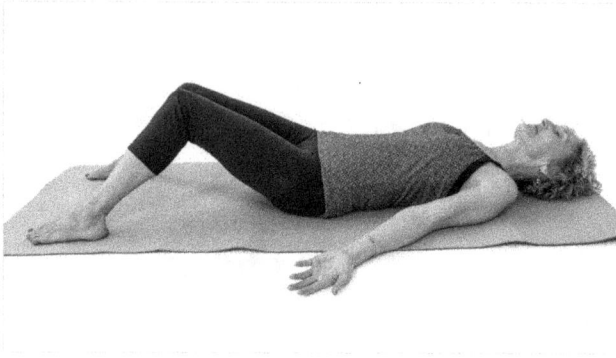

3) Spinal Release

Lay down on your back on a rug, blanket, or mat. Take a few deep breaths and relax. Bend both knees. Walk your feet away from your hips until there's a natural curve in your lower back. Now, widen your feet and rest the knees against one another. Stay here, breathing gently, for as long as you like. To sit up, roll to one side, press your hands into the floor to support the spine. as you come back up.

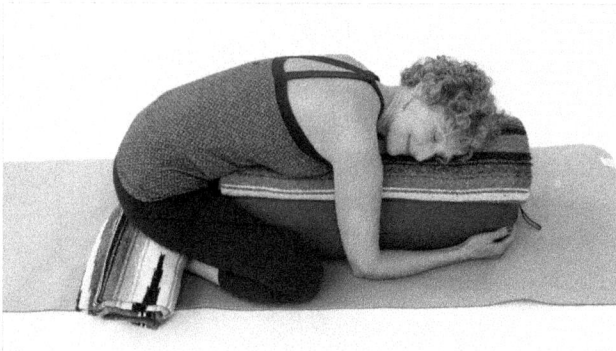

4) Lower Back Release

Kneel on the floor, with a folded blanket on your heels and a few folded blankets in between your thighs. Gently lay your chest and hips down on the blankets and relax. Stack the blankets until your body feels comfortable. Rest on one cheek, close your eyes, breathe and relax. Stay as long as you like. To lift up, press down on your hands, supporting your back with your arms.

Note: How much force do you need to apply as you hug or squeeze the legs or arms in these triage exercises? Typically, you want to match the intensity of the sensation in your body with the same amount of pressure as you hug. So, if the pain level is high, hug strongly, and if the sensation is mild, hug moderately. Never grip so hard that you stop breathing, as that is counterproductive. It may take a few tries before you figure out how hard or how gently you need to squeeze. Also note that on any given day, the amount of pressure required to reduce pain may change, so do pay attention and adjust each time you practice.

Now that we've learned a few "triage" exercises to help you get out of a challenging moment, and get back on track, let's dive into the healing power of the breath. You may be amazed to discover that specific breathing techniques can quell back pain quickly and effectively.

CHAPTER 13

BREATHE AWAY CHRONIC BACK PAIN

"Deep breathing is the greatest cure for all physical ailments." — *Edward Lankow*

In addition to correcting structural patterns of overuse, underuse, and misuse in everyday postures you can also shift pain—immediately—by improving your breath. You might not hear this from your doctor, chiropractor, or physical therapist, but it's true. The majority of people alive today misuse and underuse the breath. While it's rare that people overuse the breath by breathing too much (hyperventilation), it is very common for people to hold their breath. Inadequate breathing cannot properly nourish the cells and organs of the body.

In chapter eight, I wrote how the lack of breathing is an epidemic that undermines one's health. Under-breathing can trigger the pain response in the same way that poor posture does.

It's remarkable how many people think the best way to breathe is belly breathing, but that is only one of many, many powerful breath techniques. Imagine how boring your meals would be if you only cooked with one ingredient or ate the same food every day. Your diet would lack essential vitamins and minerals and your body would suffer. The same is true for breathing!

Different breath techniques will affect you in different ways. I cannot emphasize strongly enough that it IS absolutely possible to harness the power of your breath to facilitate healing. After decades of study and practice in the yogic and healing arts sector, I've learned how to use the breath as an effective pain management tool. I've figured out how to apply specific breathing techniques to rebalance dysfunctional patterns of misuse and underuse, to mitigate pain in my own body, and use the breath as a vital part of healthy maintenance. I teach my clients to do the same. In this chapter, I'll reveal specific

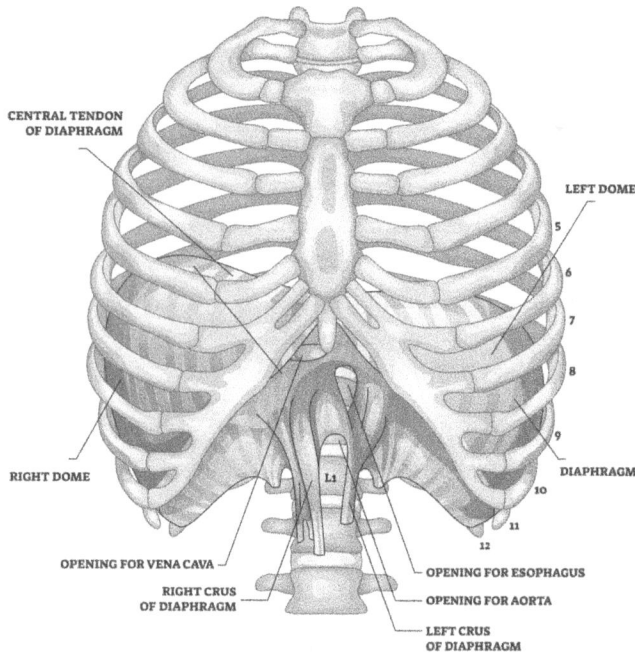

CENTRAL TENDON
OF DIAPHRAGM

LEFT DOME

5

6

7

8

9

RIGHT DOME

DIAPHRAGM

L1

10

11

12

OPENING FOR VENA CAVA

RIGHT CRUS
OF DIAPHRAGM

OPENING FOR ESOPHAGUS

OPENING FOR AORTA

LEFT CRUS
OF DIAPHRAGM

Anatomy of the Diaphragm

breath practices to correct inadequate breathing patterns and reduce chronic back pain.

Before I do, let's examine the anatomy of the breath mechanism.

At the physiological level, the respiratory organs regulate oxygen and carbon dioxide as we breathe in and out. The breath fills the blood with oxygen, nourishing the cells and repairing the tissues. The diaphragm is an umbrella-shaped muscle with two lobes that attach to the lower ribs of the rib cage on each side, forming a semi-circular pattern. The tines of the umbrella are like the ribs, expanding open as you inhale and retracting as you exhale. The lobes are anchored to the first lumbar vertebrae (L1) by two crus muscles—one on each side of the spine—which form the handle of the umbrella.

When you inhale, the diaphragm pulls down, drawing air into your lungs. When you exhale the diaphragm pushes upwards to expel air. The diaphragm is a muscle which can and must be exercised regularly to keep you strong and healthy. The breath is also a bridge between your body and spirit. So, harnessing the power of your breath is VITAL to recover from any injury or illness.

PATTERNS OF BREATHING

Humans naturally have a wide variety of breathing patterns—some healthy, some harmful. For just a moment, imagine how a baby or pet breathes—rhythmically, naturally, continually, freely. The natural unfettered breath pattern moves in and out in a continual stream of air, carrying vital energy into the body, removing waste from it. Normally, there is a momentary pause at the top and bottom of the breath as it changes direction—a pause that lasts only a second or two.

Notice how you are breathing as you read. Is your breath flowing rhythmically? Freely? Or is it bumpy and rough? Deep or shallow? Are the inhale and exhale the same length, or is one shorter? Are you holding your breath in or out? An irregular breathing pattern is common for the majority of people alive today. If your default breath does not flow in and out in an unimpeded rhythm, that, too, can contribute to physical pain. The most basic information you need to know at this stage is each inhalation can energize your body, and each exhalation can relax your body . . . if the breath flows optimally. When you're engaged in a strenuous activity, it's important to breathe deeply, vigorously. If you're trying to relax, it's better to breathe gently, slowly. As obvious as this may sound, you'd be surprised that the majority of humans do not understand the workings of their own breath, nor how to harness its power.

UNCONSCIOUS BREATHING PATTERNS

As I describe the most common unconscious breathing patterns below, try to discern which archetype is your most common "default" setting. While dysfunctional breathing patterns can create all types of mental and emotional issues, those details are beyond the scope of this book. What you can do is focus on a positive quality while you breathe in and out. Gentleness, acceptance, peace, forgiveness, compassion, etc., will send a healing message to your body.

> "
> *Humans naturally have a wide variety of breathing patterns—some healthy, some harmful.*

Common Unconscious Breathing Patterns

1) Shallow Breathing

This pattern is very common. Most people just do not breathe deeply enough. Both the inhalation and exhalation are too short to create wellbeing. The effects of shallow breathing are detrimental to the central nervous system because the cells don't receive enough oxygen. Shallow breathing can make you feel anxious, fearful, scattered, fatigued or exhausted.

2) Holding Breath IN at Top of Inhale:

At the top of the inhale, you may unconsciously hold the breath for a prolonged period before you exhale. This pattern creates anxiety in your system, as if you're bracing for the next jolt of pain. Holding the breath in is often a reaction to fear—actual or imagined—and the breath gets stuck, frozen, or shocked.

3) Holding Breath OUT at Bottom of Exhale

This pattern is also very common. You may exhale all the way out to the bottom of the breath and then hold the breath for a prolonged period before inhaling again. This chronic holding pattern can starve your whole body and all ten physiological systems of oxygen. It's a form of inadequate or under-breathing, where your body does not receive enough nourishment to heal. This pattern can give rise to feelings of sadness or depression.

4) Holding Breath IN at Top of Inhale and OUT at Bottom of Exhale

This pattern is extremely agitating to the entire system, because now you're creating two opposite dysfunctional patterns. Holding the breath both at the top and bottom disrupts the natural flow of energy into and away from you. Talk about upsetting the natural balance—it's like having anxiety and depression at the same time. Just thinking about this pattern makes my entire body ache. It can produce feelings of confusion and disorientation. When we hold our breath for chronically, or for a prolonged period, oxygen levels decrease, and carbon dioxide increases. Carbon dioxide is a soluble gas. Accumulations of it cross the blood-brain barrier and enter the bloodstream, where it lowers blood pH, making it more acidic. Acidity opens the body up to all kinds of ailments.

5) Breathing In and Out the Mouth:

"The nose is for breathing; the mouth is for eating." ~ Proverb

If your nose is stuffed up, it makes sense to breathe through the mouth, but otherwise mouth breathing is not recommended for everyday health. Breathing through the nose has many benefits which mouth breathing lacks. Cool or cold air is warmed upon entry into the body. Air particles, pollutants, dust and allergens are trapped by tiny nose hairs keeping these potential irritants out of the sinuses and the lungs. When you inhale, air passes through the blood-brain barrier, carrying vital information from the environment around you to the brain. For these reasons, nose breathing is superior to mouth breathing, but obviously, mouth breathing is better than not breathing at all.

6) Breathing IN Nose, Breathing OUT Mouth:

Breathing in through the nose and breathing out slowly through the mouth ("pffff") sounds like letting the air out of a tire. Done mindfully and consciously, this pattern acts as a stress-release valve, but done habitually or unconsciously, it inadequately nourishes the body, mind, and Spirit. A "deflated" breath can cause a defeated attitude, where you become stuck in a negative thought loop, like thinking you'll never heal.

7) Interrupted Breath:

In this pattern, either inhalation or exhalation does not flow smoothly. The inhale starts to draw in, but is immediately interrupted, so the pattern is inhale, stop, inhale, stop, etc . . . The same can occur with the exhalation. This "start-stop" pattern

> *The nose is for breathing; the mouth is for eating.*

is like river water bumping into rocks as it flows downstream. It causes turbulence. Something is preventing a smooth, deep breath from flowing in and out of your body naturally. Fear, anxiety, anger, depression, shock, or trauma are all possible reasons this pattern can occur.

I'll also mention that lackluster breathing can be caused by poor posture, where slumping of the structural body impedes the movement of the diaphragm. If you're constantly slouched over or squeezing the muscles of your back, you won't be able to enjoy a deep and nourishing breath.

RESET THE BREATH

Breath carries the beneficent life force and life force carries healing powers. The breath techniques I cover below will give you a toolkit of daily strategies to offset harm from misuse and underuse. They will help you reset dysfunctional breath patterns and establish conscious ones. It is just as important to exercise the muscle of the diaphragm as it is to strengthen any muscle. As you reestablish natural breathing patterns, chronic pain can shift within a matter of minutes. There are many positive benefits to better breathing; you'll feel more alive, your skin will glow, and your eyes will shine. An increased awareness of breath will help you select the most appropriate techniques to rebalance your specific dysfunction. Remember, your default pattern might always be the same, or it could change according to your circumstance and environment, so make sure to take note of how you are breathing in the moment before choosing a technique to practice.

For each of the techniques below follow these basic directions:

Adjust your seated position as described in "savvy sitting" on page 138. Soften and close your eyes. Turn your attention away from the sounds around you, away from the thoughts within you. Place your focus entirely on the movement of your breath. Watch the breath flow in, watch the breath flow out. Observe the breath exactly as it is in this moment.

Techniques to Correct Shallow Breathing

1) Balanced Breath I (3/3)

Take a savvy-seated position. Rest both hands on your lap or belly. Close your eyes and observe the breath. Count the length (in seconds) of your in-breath and out-breath. Notice which is longer—the inhalation or the exhalation. Over several cycles, increase the shorter half of the breath to match the longer half, until they are both the same length. For example, if your inhale is two seconds long and your exhale is three seconds, increase the inhale by one second, so both inhale and exhale last for three seconds each. Continue to breathe with this balanced rhythm for three minutes. To end the practice, relax the breath, open your eyes, and notice any changes. At this stage, it is more important to balance the inhale and exhale than it is to deepen and lengthen the breath. We'll learn to do that in the next practice.

2. Balanced Breath II (5/5)

The Heart Math Institute has done incredible research on the breath. They have proven that breathing in and out for five seconds has many health benefits. It turns on the parasympathetic nervous system (rest, digest, repair) and turns off the sympathetic nervous system (fight, flight, freeze).

Take a savvy-seated position. Place both hands on your heart, one over the other. Close your eyes and observe the breath. First, count the length of your in-breath and out-breath. Next, bring both halves of the breath into balance as you did in the first balanced breath technique. After several rounds of balanced breath, lengthen

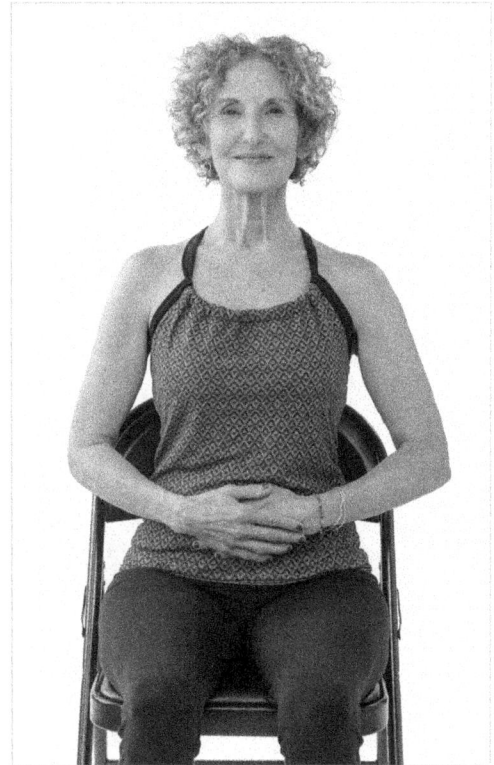

the exhalation one second by contracting your abdominal muscles and gently squeezing more breath out. Now lengthen the inhalation by one second by drawing more breath in. Both halves are still the same length, but they are both one second longer. Over several cycles, lengthen both halves of the breath again, until you reach a pattern of five seconds in and five seconds out.

Now, focus on compassion, acceptance, love or gratitude as you breathe in and out. This will balance your body, mind and emotions. Maintain this 5/5 pattern for three minutes, and then relax the breath and notice any changes in level of pain and the way you feel.

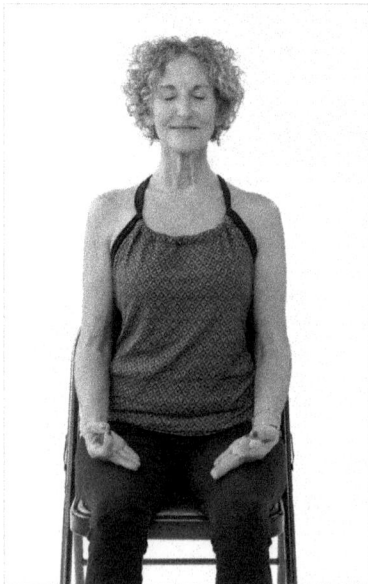

Techniques to Correct Holding the Breath

This technique will help shift patterns of holding the breath at the top, bottom, or both.

1) Circular Breath

Take a savvy-seated position. Close your eyes and observe the breath. Imagine your next inhalation moves from the space between your legs up from the base of your spine to the top of your head. Then imagine the exhalation flowing out of the top of your head back down to the base of your spine. Breathe in and draw the breath up as if it stemmed from between your legs all the way to the top of your head, and then exhale and release the breath back down to the base of the spine. Make sure when you get to the top of the inhalation to pivot the breath immediately into the exhalation, and when you get back to the bottom of the exhalation, you again pivot the breath right back into the next inhalation. Do not linger or hold the breath at the top or bottom of the breath. This will require mindful attention of the breath and a little effort to keep the breath moving in a continual circular stream of energy. Once you get the hang of this technique, practice it for three minutes and then relax and notice if there is a shift in the pattern or in the level of pain.

2) Strengthening Breath

This technique builds upon the circular breath. Here, you'll use two balls from the KA spinal rolling exercise in chapter ten. I prefer the pinky and rainbow balls as they fit nicely into the palms of the hands, but tennis balls will work, too. If you don't have two balls handy, you can make fists by wrapping the fingers around the thumbs, and gently squeeze your thumbs instead of the balls.

To begin:

Take a savvy-seated position. Hold the balls loosely in your palms, resting the back of your hands on your thighs. Close your eyes and observe the breath. Begin with the circular breathing exercise above. Once your breath is flowing freely, gently wrap all ten fingers around the balls (or tuck your thumbs into your palms and wrap your fingers around your thumbs). Either way, make sure the entire length of each finger and fingertip touches the balls (or thumbs) and the pressure of each finger on the balls (or on the thumbs) is even and steady. Squeeze your fingers gently, yet firmly enough to feel your breath deepen. Once your breath has deepened, keep the pressure steady and continue to breathe in the circular pattern—from the base of the spine, up to the top of the head, and then from the top or the head, back down, and out. Imagine it is like a fountain of energy bubbling up within you and showering you on the way out. Continue this strengthening breath practice for three minutes, and then relax your fingers slowly until the balls rest in the palms and return to a natural breath. Notice any changes.

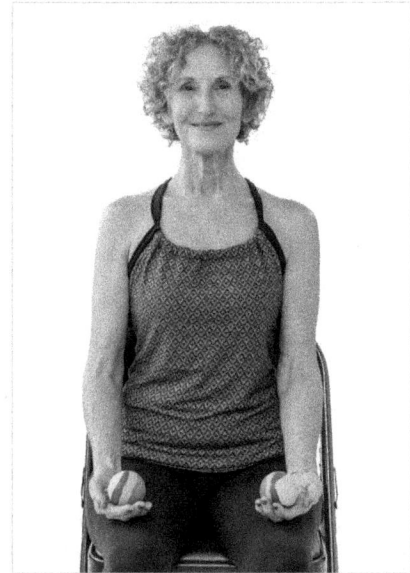

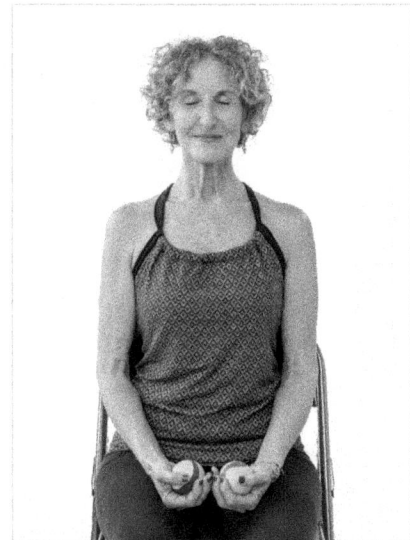

Tip: If you do not hug the balls with enough tension, your breath won't deepen. If you squeeze your fingers too tightly, you might also clench your jaw and contract the breath rather than expand it. Please be mindful of how hard you squeeze the balls, and find that sweet spot—not too loose, not too hard, just the right amount of pressure to awaken the breath.

BREATH TECHNIQUES TO REDUCE PAIN

1) Focused Breath

This technique builds upon the circular breath and the strengthening breath techniques.

To begin:

Take a savvy-seated position. Hold the balls loosely in your palms, resting the back of your hands on your thighs. Close your eyes and observe the breath. Begin with the circular breathing exercise above. Once you can maintain that, gently and firmly hug the balls (or your thumbs) with your fingers to deepen and strengthen your breath. Now, scan your back and body for the spot that registers the most sensation or pain. Focus your attention on that spot while continuing to move the breath in a circular pattern. Notice how strong the sensation feels and gently squeeze your fingers firmly to match the level of pain. Keep squeezing your fingers at that level and breathe deeply. Next, move both your attention and your breath into the area of pain. Hold your attention in that spot, breathing deeply and continually.

Imagine the inhalation bringing healing energy to the site and the exhalation dissolving and washing away sensation and pain. Continue for three minutes, and then gradually release your hands and fingers from the balls (or fists) and allow yourself to rest. Notice what has shifted.

2) Tranquility Breath (Alternate Nostril)

This breath is an excellent way to quell pain that is unpredictable and variable in frequency, intensity, and location. In the alternate breath technique, you'll bring both halves of the breath into balance, harmonizing the right and left hemispheres of the brain. This effect boosts the parasympathetic system and stimulates the Vagus nerve. The Vagus nerve controls the heart, lungs, upper digestive tract, and activates the "rest, digest and repair" mode of the central nervous system. This breath technique signals safety to your brain and body. Since there's no need for alarm, your nerves calm down and your pain dissolves. Alternate nostril breathing is truly an amazing practice. You can do this as a visualization (hand-free) or use the traditional method with the hand-position. I'll describe both variations below. Try them both and choose your favorite. The breath, as it passes through the right nostril has a warming, stimulating effect on the body and central nervous system, while the breath as it moves through the left nostril has a cooling, calming effect on the nerves making alternate nostril an excellent choice to reduce nerve pain and bring your whole system back into balance.

Tranquility Breath (Visualization)

Let's start with the visualization method. It's simple to learn and you can use it anywhere without drawing attention to yourself.

To begin:

Take a savvy-seated position, close your eyes, and balance the two halves of your breath.

Maintain an equal inhalation and exhalation. Now, imagine the exhale moves out the right nostril and down the right side of your spine to the base (tailbone), while the inhale moves from the base of the spine (tailbone) back up the right side, through the right nostril and into the center of the brow (third eye).

As you exhale, imagine the next exhale moves down from the brow, through the left nostril, to the base of the spine. As you breathe back in, visualize the breath flowing from the base back, up the left side of the spine, through the left nostril, and into the brow.

As you continue to breathe, you change sides at the space of the brow. Down the right, up the right. Down the left, up the left. Continue for three minutes and then return to a natural breath. Notice how your mind, breath, body, and back are feeling now. Do you feel more centered? Has stress melted away? Has pain diminished?

Tranquility Breath (Traditional)

The traditional method is more advanced than the hands-free method. Repeat the instructions for the visualization method above, but instead of imaging the breath flowing up one side and down the other side, you'll use your fingers to guide the breath.

To begin:

Repeat the instructions for the hand-free method. Place your right thumb lightly on the curl of the right nostril, rest the index and middle finger on the brow, and place your ring finger lightly on the curl of the left nostril. The pinky finger extends away from your face.

Once you reach the top of the inhalation, press the ring finger against the left nostril (closing the passageway), and exhale from the brow, down the right side, to the base of the spine. Inhale back up the right side.

When you get to the top of this breath, release the ring finger to open the left nostril, press the thumb to close off the right nostril, and exhale down and up the left side.

Keep going back and forth, using your fingers to open the nostril on the side the breath is flowing in or out of, while keeping the other nostril closed until it's time to switch sides. Once you become comfortable with alternate nostril breathing, you can extend the length of each inhale and each exhale to five seconds or more.

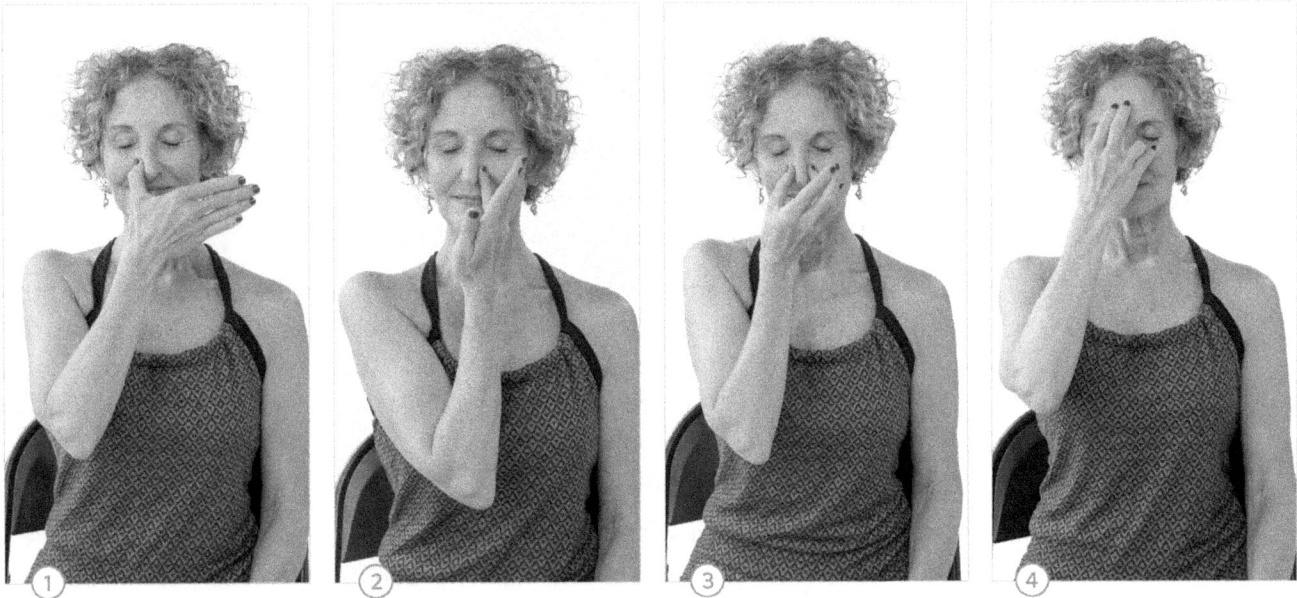

Tranquility Breath

Continue alternate nostril breathing for three minutes. Then, release your hand, sit quietly, and breathe naturally. Notice the effects of this technique on your body, mind, and Spirit. How are you feeling now?

3. Moon Breath (Soothing)

This breath is only half of the alternate nostril breath. Using moon breath, you block off the right nostril and breathe in and out of the left nostril. The left channel is soothing and cooling and calming to the body, so use the moon breath to alleviate sharp fiery nerve pain.

With this technique, it is best to use the hand placement (instead of the visualization method) because it channels all of the breath through the left nostril, making it more effective.

To begin:
Take a savvy-seated position. Close your eyes and focus your attention to the breath. Balance the inhale and exhale and extend to four or five counts in length.

You can visualize this pattern or use the hand position.

Next, place your right thumb over the right nostril, index and middle fingers on the brow, and leave the ring and pinky fingers floating freely.

As you exhale, close off the right nostril and keep the left nostril open. Send the breath down the left side to the base of your spine. Inhale back up the left side to the brow. Exhale from the brow, back down the left side, to the base. Continue breathing up/in and down/out ONLY through the left nostril to calm and soothe your nervous system. After three minutes, relax your hand and return to natural breathing. Notice how you feel now.

4) Cooling Breath: (Relaxes the Nerves)

This breath is cooling in nature and will help quell any intense pain or burning sensations in your body or back. It mimics the action of sipping a cool liquid through a straw. There are two mouth positions—traditional and modified. You need to be able to curl your tongue for the first one. If you cannot curl your tongue, use the modified position.

Traditional

Take a savvy-seated position, close your eyes, and focus on the flow of the breath. Allow your mouth to fill up with saliva. When it does, open your mouth, stick out your tongue and curl it up like a hollow tube. Suck air in through the tube, making a slurpy sound. When you run out of air, swallow. Repeat 5–10 times. The air rushing over the saliva helps to cool and calm the brain and nerves.

Modified

If you cannot curl your tongue, no problem. Repeat the same instructions, this time purse your lips into a round shape and suck the air in through your lips and over the saliva—it will work just as well.

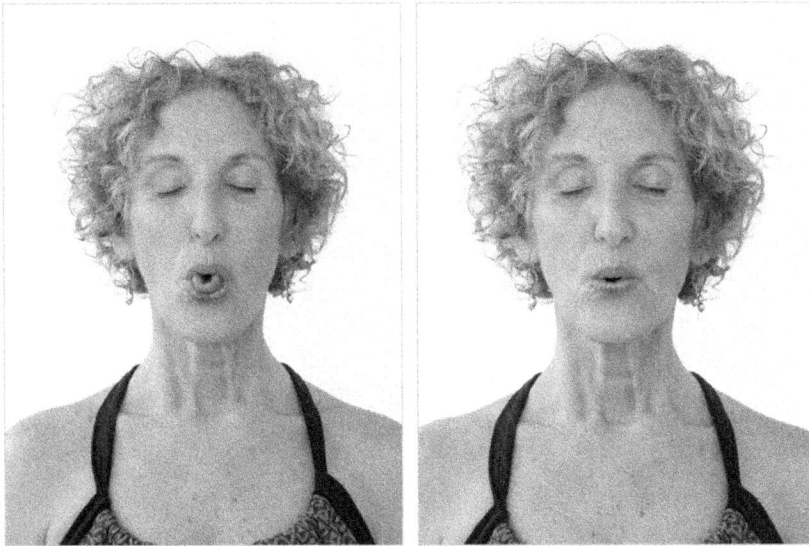

Cooling Breath

5) Bellows Breath (Invigorating)

Back pain from underuse and inactivity is often dull, sore and achy. This pain typically radiates from the same spot—lower back, sacrum, neck, etc. It never gets worse, nor completely goes away. Usually this type of pain arises from under-activity and responds well to aligned movement. Because this pain arises from too little activity, the bellows breath stimulates the breath, and increases healthy flow of blood and lymph. Bellows breath is moderately paced, measured in rhythm, and steady out and in. Using it, you contract the diaphragm muscle in short bursts, breathing out and in through the nose, with lips closed and teeth relaxed. The breath starts with the exhale. The rhythm of this breath is similar to the speed of pumping a bellows to ignite a spark of fire from cool embers in a fireplace or woodstove.

To begin:

Take a savvy-seated position. Close your eyes and focus your attention to the breath. Place one hand on your solar plexus so you can feel the diaphragm pulse in and out as you breathe. Place the other palm in front of your nose, about 2–3 inches away, so you can feel each exhale. This hand position will help you observe the pace of the breath moving in and out. Once you are comfortable with this, you can place your hands on your thighs or cup them in your lap. With your lips closed, take one deep breath IN to prepare. As you exhale, pull the upper abdominals back towards the spine to contract the diaphragm, and immediately release the abdominal muscles to create a short, steady, in/out rhythm. Puff the breath out through the nose for one second and back in through the nose for one second. Don't go faster or slower; try to maintain a one-two rhythm. Continue until you've run out of breath. Take another deep breath in and repeat two more cycles, for a total of three rounds. You'll feel more blood and energy circulating inside you. Notice if your awareness of pain has shifted.

6) Balanced Breath with Retention (Nourishing)

I love this four part breath to balance my mind, hormones, and emotions. It feels so nourishing and always leaves me with the perfect blend of energy and calm—what I call "centered." In a centered state, your mind is alert and relaxed, you are not reacting to outside stimuli, and can simply enjoy the depth of your own "being." Ahhhh!

The pattern is: inhale for four counts, hold for four counts, exhale for four counts, and hold for four counts. The hold is called breath retention. This is a purposeful and mindful practice, unlike the dysfunctional pattern of unconsciously holding the breath to avoid unpleasant situations or to react to outside stimuli. Retention of the in-breath allows your blood time to absorb increased amounts of oxygen. Retention of the out-breath allows your blood to dump more carbon dioxide. This is an efficient form of respiration that can put you into a "feel good" state.

To begin:

Take a savvy seat. Soften and close your eyes. Turn your attention away from sounds around you, away from the thoughts within you, and focus on the sound and movement of your own breath. Staying quiet and still, notice your natural breath. Which half is longer—your inhale or exhale? Notice how long each cycle is. Silently count how many seconds your inhalation lasts and how many seconds your exhalation lasts.

Gently lengthen the shorter half to equal the longer half. Now both halves of your breath are in balance—the same length. Keep breathing in and out evenly, gently, and kindly. Now, set the meter to four breaths in and four breaths out.

Note: It's also fine to use 3/3, 5/5, or even 6/6, but I wouldn't recommend more than 6/6. Every time you practice, choose whichever count you feel most comfortable with in that moment.

Once you're comfortable with your chosen rhythm, add a "hold" to the top, and later add another "hold" to the bottom.

Begin like this:
Breathe IN for four counts, hold the breath for four counts, and breathe out for four counts. Repeat.

Note: Practice this pattern several times (even several days) to get comfortable with holding the breath IN at the top of the inhale, BEFORE you add the retention at the bottom of the exhalation.

Once you are comfortable with the first pattern, add the retention at the base of the exhale. The full pattern goes like this: Breathe IN for four counts, hold the breath in for four counts, breath out for four counts, hold the breath out for four counts. Repeat the full cycle for three minutes. Relax and observe how you feel.

Tips: If you are new to breathing techniques, practice the In-4, Out-4 breath for a week. The following week, add the first retention at the top of the inhalation (In-4, Hold-4, Out-4) until you're comfortable with that. The third week, you can add the second retention at the base of the exhalation (In-4, Hold-4, Out-4, Hold-4). Remember, these are techniques that you can use for the rest of your life to get out of pain and to stay out of pain. When you are retaining the breath, hold it gently without cringing or tensing your muscles. Imagine you are holding something precious and valuable, because you are—the breath!

PAIN-BE-GONE TECHNIQUE

Pain is a common experience for all people. It's part of life. One that can shift for the better or for the worse. When you harness the healing power of your breath, you can use it to dissolve pain. This focused exercise requires a willingness to enter into the sensation rather than retracting from it. As you focus on the exact spot where pain resides and remain attentive to the sensation by breathing into it and releasing it, in time, it will change. Because you're finally paying attention to pain with an attitude of openness and compassion, pain will start to dissolve. I've seen huge results within the span of several minutes of concentrated focus. Just remember, do not identify with "my" pain, just be aware of a sensation "of" pain.

To begin:
Take a savvy-seated position. Close your eyes and place your attention fully on the breath. Bring the inhalation and exhalation into equal balance and rhythm and breathe this way for a minute or two. Now, scan your body from head to toe. Notice all the places where you experience a sensation of unrest, discomfort, or pain. Identify which area is in the most distress, and fix your attention on this area as you continue breathing rhythmically. Scan the general area up-and-down, and side-to-side. Is there a single spot where you feel the most pain? If not, stay focused on the general area. If so, focus on that singular spot. Keep breathing and stay with the sensation of pain.

Next, move your attention INTO the sensation of pain—do not run away from it. Draw each inhalation directly into the general area or single spot of pain and imagine the breath infusing the spot with healing energy. As you exhale, imagine and allow the sensation of pain to dissolve.

Sometimes, pain simply dissolves after a few minutes. Other times, pain moves to another location. If this happens, move your attention and breath to the new location and repeat the instructions above. If the pain moves again, keep following it wherever it goes, until it disappears. Rarely does this technique fail to work if you approach yourself and your experience of pain with genuine compassion, love, acceptance, and forgiveness.

PART THREE CONCLUSION

Now you know many different breathing techniques that can improve your habitually inadequate breathing patterns! Perhaps you've realized the connection between poor posture and optimal alignment, lackluster breathing, and optimal breath. When you adjust your physical posture, your breath will naturally begin to improve. And, when you also start to breathe deeply and consciously, you can reduce chronic back pain and speed the healing process. Posture and breathing go together like a hand and a glove. The patterns described above are just a handful of all the techniques I know, practice, and love to teach to maintain health and wellbeing.

Start slowly and build up a repertoire of useful breathing and alignment practices over time. You will find your favorite "go-to" practices. Then, once you are out of pain, you, too, can use these practices to keep you out of pain.

If you need additional support to successfully integrate these new habits, checkout *The BackCare Blueprint* online video companion course.

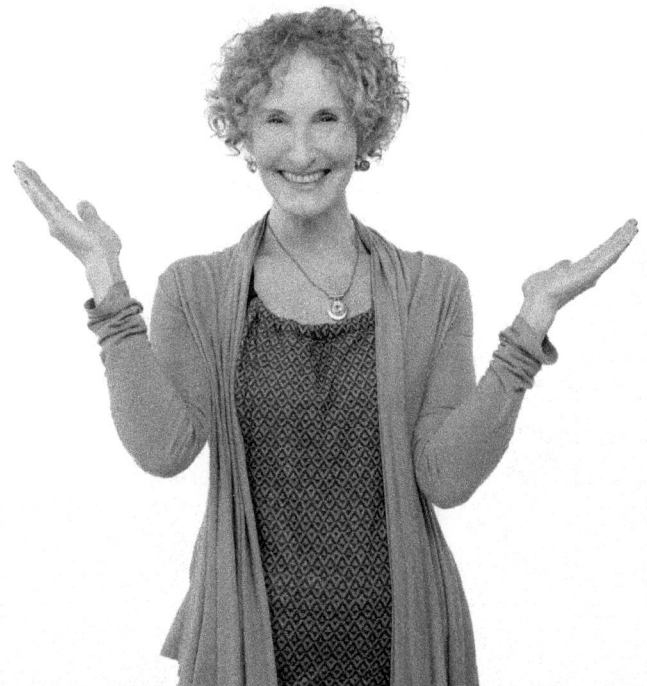

CONCLUSION

Congratulations for taking a very important step on the road to recovery! By reading this book and considering the new ideas contained herein, you now know a lot more about addressing chronic back pain and improving spinal health yourself!

To get this far, you had to evaluate the magnitude of an astounding scientific statistic:

75% of all back pain is caused by structural misalignment and poor posture. You wrestled with the reality that few doctors ever mention this statistic, much less teach their patients how to improve spinal health. You now see how the fact that most people don't know how to properly care for their back is no real fault of their own. And you understand that the current back-pain epidemic is indicative of a modern culture that does not fully grasp or appreciate the intelligent design, function, and power of the human body. You've learned how that is symptomatic of a medical system designed to keep people ignorant of the innate self-healing power, one that tethers patients to a treadmill of "Done-For-You" mechanistic treatment, instead of providing a pathway towards a "Done-With-You" or a "Do-It-Yourself" model of sustainable healthcare. In addition, you now know that the widespread occurrence of back pain arises from an overly sedentary lifestyle, resulting in 21st century syndromes such as sitter's disease and text neck. So, it's no wonder you've been stuck with pain, the deck has been stacked against you!

I hope you understand how chronic misalignment, lackluster breathing, and negative mindset have contributed to chronic imbalances in your body that landed you in this predicament—trapped in a cycle of chronic back pain, book in hand, looking for a way out! Certainly, you've become aware of what's missing in your current approach to back pain management—YOU! And you've experienced firsthand how structural imbalances trigger the pain response. Hopefully, you've discovered that

> ❝
> *You've become aware of what's missing in your current approach to back pain management— YOU!*

pain is really an ally—the primary messenger that draws attention, warns you when something is amiss, and signals you to take corrective measures. However, because pain muddles one's thoughts and disrupts one's emotions, it can be a challenge to know which choices to make to improve your spinal health. And in those moments, when back pain has flared up, it's *The BackCare Blueprint* to the rescue.

Remember, *The BackCare Blueprint*, by design and necessity, is an integrated holistic method that puts you in the driver's seat of your own recovery and of your future health. By your own willingness to identify postural and structural causes of chronic back pain and become an active participant in the healing process, you can chart a new pathway forward. One of self-awareness, where you know which alignment and breath practices to use to mitigate pain, and a self-reliant approach where you create and sustain spinal health and wellness instead of masking its symptoms. A lifestyle where you heal and thrive!

So, what do you do now about your situation?

First, make the connection between chronically poor postural habits, lackluster breathing, negative attitudes, and chronic back pain. Since posture, breath, and mindset are only under your immediate control, not anyone else's, it's obvious that learning to correct structural misalignment, enhance the breath, and engender mental positivity are all excellent strategies that you can use every day on your own behalf. Speaking from personal and professional experience, I'd say these are the most effective ways to relieve chronic back pain and without the negative side effects of pills, shots, and surgery.

Next, identify your "cocktail pose" and begin to study your habits. Notice when and how your spine is out of alignment, discern which postural habits cause pain, and adjust your body accordingly, using the biomechanical principles presented herein.

> "
> Remember,
> The BackCare
> Blueprint, *by
> design and
> necessity, is
> an integrated
> holistic method
> that puts you
> in the driver's
> seat of your own
> recovery and
> of your future
> health.*

The simple act of doing something for yourself will have an immediate and positive impact on your spinal health. Then, notice your breathing habits and attitude defaults and make adjustments there, too. Once you instill healthy habits consistently over time, you will stimulate the self-healing mechanism of your body and break free from the debilitating cycle of chronic back pain. By following *The BackCare Blueprint* approach, you will eventually shift from the "Done-For-You" medical model (which requires no participation in the healing process other than showing up for appointments) to the "Do-It-Yourself" method, where you become self-empowered and self-reliant with your spinal self-care.

Follow the practical tips, listed on the next page, and start *The BackCare Blueprint* program today!

Once you develop a spinal self-care routine, you'll feel so much better. Chronic back pain will dissolve, joy will surface, and you'll feel like your wonderful self again.

In case you've forgotten the healthy person hidden inside the one who's in pain, let's conclude this book by returning to your personal vision of health.

Imagine yourself enjoying an activity that you love to do—without any pain! What are you doing? Are you playing with others or by yourself? Are you smiling? What aspects of your life feel inspired? How are you spending your free time now that you're not running from doctor to specialist, from one appointment to another? How have your relationships improved? How has your ability to work and play shifted? Do you experience greater ease and more freedom? Do you feel relieved? Happy? Energized?

When you decide to take *The BackCare Blueprint* program to heart and dive into the practices, I would love to hear your success story. Then, you can join the ranks of people like Mark, Laura, Marjorie, John, Rani, Jane, Nan, and so many others who've learned how to get themselves out of pain and how to keep themselves out of pain.

TIPS FOR GETTING STARTED WITH THE BACKCARE BLUEPRINT

- Make a commitment today to improve spinal self-care.

- Schedule time in your main calendar, daily, to practice the exercises.

- Every day, revisit your vision of health and affirm that your back is improving.

- Use the KA ball rolling every day—trust me, within a few days you'll be hooked!

- Begin with the self-traction exercise and use it throughout the day.

- Practice one technique for a week, and when you've gotten the hang of it, learn the next.

- Do a short routine (5–15 minutes) at the same time every day, if possible.

- Once you're familiar with all the practices, use the ones that work best for you.

- Heed your body's warning signals. Get up and move as soon as your back starts to feel stiff. Don't wait until you're in a lot of pain to take corrective actions.

- Check out the companion online video course, especially if you're a visual learner.

- Contact me for 1:1 support if you really get stuck. I'm here to help you!

PART FOUR

ADDITIONAL RESOURCES

Part Four provides information for those who wish to substitute natural medicines and herbal remedies for pharmaceutical pain medications. If you're currently taking high doses of any medicine, consult your doctor and let them know of your decision to wean off them. They can provide recommendations for how to best reach your goal. What follows are effective and affordable plant-based remedies in the form of creams, essential oils, tinctures and more. I hope they help you as much as they have helped (and still help) me to live a pain-free life.

HERBAL ALLIES

When clients initially sought my assistance, most had been taking pharmaceutical painkillers for a long time. They all wanted to stop relying on pills, so I suggested they try herbal remedies for pain relief instead. The products discussed below are herbal plant medicines and effective remedies for pain that have no detrimental or negative side effects. None! If you wish to wean off prescription or over-the-counter pain medications, start using these herbal allies immediately to help you transition. You can use these herbal remedies for as long as you need. I always keep Arnica and Rescue Remedy in my medicine cabinet. These products provide significant pain relief without negative side effects, but remember they won't remove the cause of back pain if that cause is from a structural misalignment (or disease). You'll still need to adjust your physical alignment and create pain-free postural habits. However, these herbal remedies make a great substitute for both prescription and over-the-counter painkillers and come in handy for those times when you're unable to improve your posture and alleviate pain on your own, and they are a wonderful companion to any treatment—safe for everyday use!

> Herbal remedies make a great substitute for both prescription and over-the-counter painkillers.

Herbal plant medicines come in many forms: creams, gels, balms, salves, tinctures, pellets, tablets, drops, and concentrated essential oils. They can be applied topically, ingested orally, inhaled, or added to a steam, diffuser, or bath. Oral medicines, whether allopathic or herbal, must traverse the digestive tract and be assimilated before their active components are released into the bloodstream and made available for pain relief.

Homeopathic medicines work with the understanding that "less is more." In the form of pellets, tablets, or drops, these remedies are dissolved under the tongue where they enter the bloodstream directly—within seconds—impacting the body much faster than ordinary painkillers that are swallowed and digested before being absorbed. Topical homeopathic creams and gels applied directly on the skin, quickly deliver their active components to the affected tissues. Applying essential oils dermally is an incredibly effective method to provide healing directly to the site of an injury, or location of pain. Within seconds, essential oils and herbs are absorbed into the skin, quickly reducing pain and inflammation to promote healing. When inhaled, essential oils can cross the blood brain barrier, immediately interacting with pain receptors, neurons, and the pain messaging system of the brain. All of these medicines and methods—whether ingested, inhaled, or topically applied—can deliver relief faster than swallowing a pill, waiting for it to digest, and then circulate through the bloodstream to the affected area.

FAVORITES

Arnica—cream, gel, tablets, pellets, drops

Arnica is an herbal homeopathic remedy used for trauma, muscle pain and stiffness, swelling from injury, and discoloration from bruising. It is made from the botanical plant, 'arnica montana', which is one of the most effective natural pain relief plant remedies that exists. This homeopathic medicine is available in several forms—topical cream and gel, oral tablet, pellet, or drops. The cream and gel are for external use only, so do not use them on open wounds, around the eyes, nostrils, anus, or vaginal areas where the skin is thin and tender. The difference in efficacy between cream and gel is negligible—it's really a matter of preference. Topicals are applied by rubbing liberally onto the site of pain as often as needed. Orals are more convenient if the affected area requires removing clothing to apply (such as your sacrum or lower back). The orals have recommended dosages on the package and should be followed. Make sure you never touch the homeopathic tablets or pellets with your fingers. Hold the cap upside down and twist once for one pellet, twice for two pellets, etc. Then, open your mouth and pop the pellets under your tongue without touching. Tablets have a twist-off cap, so shake as many as you need into the cap, and then pop them under your tongue. Allow them to dissolve without chewing, that way the herbs enter into the bloodstream directly to provide quick relief.

I prefer to use homeopathic orals at the onset of injury and for acute pain—for those times when you tweak your back by twisting to reach something in the back seat of your car or by bending abruptly to pick something up. I typically use creams and gels for ongoing low-grade sensations. Also, orals are great when pain sensations cover a large area, and topicals when pain is localized.

Potencies vary, so it's important to know that lower potencies (6C or 6X) are best for chronic issues and higher potencies (30X—200C) are best for acute conditions. If you have an acute injury, you might start with one dose of the higher potency (200C), and then switch to the lower range (30C or 30X) as your body heals. Lower potencies can be taken every few hours, whereas high potencies might be taken only once a week. Most stores provide a chart to help you select the proper potency, but you can also seek guidance from a homeopath.

> 66
>
> **arnica montana** *is one of the most effective natural pain relief plant remedies that exists.*

Traumeel

Traumeel is another excellent homeopathic remedy for minor muscle and joint pain caused by sprain, strain, and bruising. Packaged most commonly in a tube as a topical cream or gel, it is also available in tablets. Traumeel combines fourteen herbal plants that provide multi-targeted restoration of balance—it can reduce pain, swelling, soreness, bruising, and minor bleeding. Traumeel stimulates immune function, enhances healing, and is a wonderful analgesic and anti-inflammatory aid for all types of joint pain and arthritis. For topical use, apply liberally as needed. For oral use, follow the recommendations provided.

Rescue Remedy

Another type of natural plant remedy is called a flower essence. Flower essences are used for everyday situations to bring the body, mind, and emotions back into balance. Flower essences or flower remedies are infusions made from the flowering part of a plant. Unlike essential oils or herbal teas, which use the flower, leaf and/or stem to make an herbal medicine, a flower essence does not contain any physical part of the plant. The process involves steeping the flower in water, under sunlight or moonlight, and capturing the energy imprint of the plant and infusing the water with its healing vibration. Rescue Remedy, created by the Bach Flower Remedy company, is a combination of five flower essences: impatiens, star of Bethlehem, cherry plum, rock rose, and clematis. It is often used for acute pain and severe trauma, in emergency and crisis situations. It is effective for any stressful situation as it helps to counter fear and anxiety, promote physical relaxation, emotional calm, and mental focus. There are several single flower essences that are equally effective in reducing physical pain such as sweet chestnut, gorse, gentian, walnut, heather and holly. And while the Bach Flower Remedy company is famous for their Rescue Remedy, there are many excellent flower essence companies on the market.

Essential Oils

Essential oils are concentrated forms of plant material effective for relieving all types of pain. They penetrate the skin quickly, and are rapidly absorbed, providing nutrients, oxygen (through increased circulation), and beneficial anti-inflammatory agents to your most painful areas. It's safe to use essential oils right out of the bottle, but since these plant medicines are very concentrated, it's best to add several drops to a liquid "base" oil, such as olive, almond, coconut, or sesame oil before applying to the skin. This is especially true for any citrus essential oils, as they can burn tender skin when directly applied in undiluted form. Essential oils are most commonly used topically for pain relief. In some cases, they may be used internally (a few drops in water), but extra care must be taken depending on the type and strength of the specific oil that you are ingesting. For the purposes of this book, I'll suggest topical use. Equally effective is inhaling essential oils. The scents can calm or invigorate, thus stimulating your brain to send a soothing message to your body. You may also add several drops to a hot bath or an infuser/steamer to soothe or stimulate yourself depending on what you need in order to come back into balance.

TOP 15 ESSENTIAL OILS FOR PAIN RELIEF (LISTED ALPHABETICALLY)

Chamomile is an effective anti-inflammatory and antispasmodic agent, good for lower back pain, muscular pain, and neuralgia, among other uses.

Copaiba reduces nerve pain and lessens neuropathy, reduces muscle spasms and muscle pain, and relieves arthritis.

Eucalyptus helps heal muscular aches, sprains, strains, and nerve pain.

Frankincense is the "King of Oils." It has an incredible fragrance and reduces chronic muscle pain, arthritic pain, and nerve pain.

Ginger is an analgesic that provides pain relief by acting on vanilloid receptors, which are located on sensory nerve endings. Ginger extract could be substituted for NSAID's (non-steroidal anti-inflammatory drugs). It's great for anyone dealing with a lot of pain.

Helichrysum is an effective antispasmodic, analgesic, and anti-inflammatory, and is great for muscle bruising, and tension, and heals the skin after sunburn.

Holy Basil is an analgesic, antidepressant, and antispasmodic. It's useful for calming nerve pain including sciatic nerve pain and for stimulating the nerves when numbness occurs.

Juniper Berry relieves muscle spasms, joint and muscle aches from arthritis, fibromyalgia, and nerve pain.

Lavender is the most common essential oil, as it soothes tension, stress, anxiety and reduces nerve pain.

Myrrh is full of terpenoids and sesquiterpenes, which have anti-inflammatory and antioxidant properties. Myrrh is more effective when combined with frankincense.

Palo Santo has a rich supply of antioxidants and terpenes, including natural limonene and alpha-terpineol. It is used for arthritis, injuries, and chronic back or neck pain.

Peppermint is an anti-inflammatory, can relax tense or achy muscles, and soothe nerve pain.

Rosemary contains rosmarinic acid, which relieves achy muscles, joints, rheumatism, and nerve pain.

Spruce is rich in monoterpenes, which give this oil anti-inflammatory and analgesic powers. Great for joint pain.

Wintergreen is an anti-inflammatory and analgesic, alleviating muscle and bone pain and reducing discomfort in the joints.

Ylang Ylang effectively facilitates the healing of wounds, enhances the health of the nervous system, reduces the stress exerted on the nerves, balances blood pressure levels, and stabilizes the heart rate.

At the height of sciatic pain, I went to bed holding a bottle of ylang ylang to my nose. Breathing in this healing oil for about twenty minutes would calm my nerves enough so I could fall asleep. It was a lifesaver for me!

Trauma Oil Blend: Arnica, St John's Wort, Calendula—in a base oil—relieves swelling in the joints, muscle spasms, nerve pain, and arthritis. It heals muscles, ligaments, tendons, bruises, and can alleviate headaches. You can also add a few drops of any essential oil from the list above to the trauma oil and create your own personal blend.

Most stores have display bottles which allow you to smell any essential oil before purchase. This is a great way to discover which oils are right for you. Close your eyes, hold the bottle a few inches from your nose and breathe in its scent. Then notice how you react. Does the fragrance stimulate or calm you? Does your body say "yes" or "no" to the fragrance? Purchase the ones that agree with your system.

TURMERIC

Turmeric is one of the best anti-inflammatory plants in the world. Turmeric contains the active compound, curcumin, which inhibits an inflammatory cytokine involved in rheumatoid arthritis. Turmeric has also been proven to work as well as, if not better than, conventional over-the- counter painkillers, like ibuprofen. Look for capsules that contain powder made from the whole turmeric root, not from an extract of curcumin, because the whole plant contains many healing agents other than curcumin. It should also contain piperine (pepper) which boosts the efficacy of the turmeric. Take turmeric daily, or as needed, because reducing inflammation reduces pain.

CBD

The cannabis plant has been used for over 5,000 years for its fiber, oil, and medicinal properties. Before the 1900s, almost all the world's bibles, maps, sails, clothes and books were from cannabis fiber. Hemp has over 50,000 commercial uses including medicine, paper, food, rope, nets, lace, soap, shoes, plastics, explosives, caulking, fiberboard, paint, sealant, methanol, gasoline, bricks, charcoal, auto bodies, packing, lubricants, oil for fuel and lighting, animal feed, furniture, mats, varnish, lotions, ointments, lacquer, and salad dressings.

In 1970, the US Federal Government classified marijuana as a Schedule 1 drug (with a high potential for abuse) as part of the war on drugs campaign and made it illegal in all fifty states.

Fortunately, as research was conducted and health benefits of cannabis again became recognized, more states and countries have decriminalized and legalized cannabis, allowing increased access to its healing benefits. As of this writing, thirty-eight US states have legalized cannabis for medicinal use including Alaska, Arizona, Arkansas, California, Colorado, Connecticut, Delaware, District of Columbia, Florida, Hawaii, Illinois, Kansas, Louisiana, Maine, Maryland, Massachusetts, Michigan, Minnesota, Mississippi, Missouri, Montana, Nevada, New Hampshire, New Jersey, New Mexico, New York, North Dakota, Ohio, Oklahoma, Oregon, Pennsylvania, Rhode Island, South Carolina, Utah, Vermont, Virginia, Washington, and West Virginia. That number continues to rise, but the US federal government lags and still classifies marijuana as a Schedule 1 drug.

Cannabis has three medicinal components: cannabinoids, terpenoids, and flavonoids. While there are over 113 known cannabinoids, these two are the most important: tetrahydrocannabinol (THC) and cannabidiol (CBD). CBD was discovered back in 1940, and unlike THC, it has no psychoactive effects, meaning it will not get

> **CBD, as an oral product, has been proven to reduce chronic back pain, nerve pain, and arthritic pain caused by inflammation.**

you high. The body of modern scientific research of cannabis continues to grow and one of the proven benefits is pain reduction.

A meta-analysis published in 2017 looked at twenty-four different clinical trials involving 1,334 patients over several years and demographics. These studies used various forms of cannabis for treating chronic pain and the results showed up to a 50% reduction in chronic pain.

CBD, as an oral product, has been proven to reduce chronic back pain, nerve pain, and arthritic pain caused by inflammation. CBD can help injuries heal faster because cannabinoids have anti-inflammatory and neuroprotective properties that relieve pain and improve regeneration.

CBD can be purchased—where legal—as a topical cream, oral tincture, capsule, spray, patch, smoke, vape, culinary oil or edible. CBD offers antioxidant support and relieves muscle tension and inflammation. It stimulates the endocannabinoid system (ECS) of the body, interacting with CB1 receptors in the neurons of the brain responsible for regulating inflammatory pain transmission and with the CB2 receptors in the immune cells, which reduce inflammation in the gut and bowels. CBD works well for some people, but not for others, so it's worth finding out if CBD will help you.

Most people do not know that the human body naturally produces endo-cannabinoids, which are structurally similar to cannabinoid molecules of the cannabis plant. Both human endocannabinoids and plant cannabinoids can activate the CB1 and CB2 receptors of the brain to manage pain naturally. The first endocannabinoid discovered was named "anandamide" after the Sanskrit word "Ananda" or bliss. Every human has cannabis-like molecules floating around in their brain and this is partly why mind-body techniques like the ones I taught you in Part Three actually work to mitigate pain.

Here is a brief introduction to the variety of CBD products available followed by a list of criteria for selecting high-quality products containing active potent ingredients because the market is flooded with many low-quality cannabis products.

CBD Potency

Typically, the higher the potency, the more efficacious the product. Potency is rarely an issue with topical products, but with oral CBD products it's often recommended to start with a lower dose and increase potency over time to find what works best for you. The size and mass of your body is a factor, as is your sensitivity to how well and how quickly CBD will work for you. Some people need high doses of CBD to feel any pain relief, while others only need low doses to experience the benefits. If you are in considerable pain, you might very well need a higher dose. Just realize the higher the potency, the higher the price tag. CBD products, by law, contain less than .03% THC, so you won't get high from any of them.

Tinctures for General Pain

Tinctures are an oral form, where concentrated CBD is blended with a base oil. Tinctures are available flavored or unflavored. Fruit flavored tinctures are popular because they mask the "musky" taste of marijuana. Potencies vary widely, ranging between 100 mg–7,500mg per 30ml/bottle. That's a huge difference, but one benefit of starting with a lower potency is that you won't spend as much money. Do some research and go with your intuition (or pocketbook) on which potency to begin with, or purchase products in a dispensary store (instead of online) where you can speak with a trained salesperson about which dosage might be best for your situation.

Topicals for Localized Pain

Creams, lotions, salves, balms, patches, and massage oils are applied liberally to the site of localized pain, as often as needed. Standard potency is typically anywhere from 200–750mg per jar, or 3–8 mg per application, or 50mg/tsp up to 50mg/tbsp, depending on the product. Some products contain as little as 0.5mg/ml, so buyer beware. You get what you pay for: the higher the potency, the greater the price. A low potency (20–100 mg/ml) topical might not provide any relief. Medium potency (200–700 mg/ml topicals are perfect for muscle soreness, strain, sprain, bruising. Higher potencies (700–4,000/mg/ml) are good for neuropathic pain. Topicals are most handy when your back pain occurs in a specific area that you can easily access. If you cannot reach an area with your hand (like the mid-back), orals may be a better choice for you.

Orals/Edibles for General Pain

Tinctures and soft gel capsules are the most popular forms of CBD for medicinal oral use. And most are helpful for relieving general pain and nerve pain. Some people prefer edibles like gummies or chocolate to relax and calm the whole nervous system. Personally, I prefer the purity of oral tinctures because the edibles contain added sugars, which can negatively impact one's immune system and impede healing. Start with no more than 50mg per day and go up from there. A standard oral dose is 20mg/ml and high dose is 50mg/ml. Bear in mind that tinctures act quickly, and you could feel relief in about thirty minutes. Soft gels are typically found in potencies of 25–50 mg per dose and take a bit longer to activate since the capsule must dissolve before the CBD is released. Edibles take the longest to act, as they must pass through the digestive tract before being absorbed into the blood.

Product Criteria

No matter which type of CBD product you choose, you'll want to buy a quality product. These recommendations will guide you.

- Full-spectrum hemp extracts that provide the widest array of cannabinoids and terpenes, over broad-spectrum extracts, or CBD isolates.
- Third-party lab testing to ensure accurate potency and purity from heavy metals, mycotoxins, pesticides, herbicides. *testing for over 200 common contaminants.
- Companies that list the test results on their website.
- Organically grown non-GMO hemp products.
- Companies that disclose the source of their hemp. Oregon, Colorado, Alabama, Canada and Scandinavia have high standards for cultivation and clean soils.
- Products extracted with supercritical CO_2. Do not buy products that use solvents like ethanol, methanol, hexane, ether or butane to extract the CBD. CO_2 is harmless, and as soon as pressure is released, the CO_2 gas evaporates completely, leaving no harmful chemical residues.
- Companies that offer a satisfaction guarantee.
- Companies that have transparency and provide details on each stage of production listed on their website.
- Companies that have a reputable customer service.
- Products based on your taste or scent preference.
- Products based on your finances.

Note: As with any medicine, natural or synthetic, it is important to ensure that an herbal remedy will not interfere with any medication you are currently taking. Please check with your medical team or doctor for such advice.

As popular as CBD has become in recent years, the other herbal medicines mentioned above are much less expensive. If you're new to plant medicines, start with tried-and-true topicals, like Traumeel and arnica. If they don't work, try essential oils, and if you still need relief, you might experiment with CBD. If you tweak your back, immediately take arnica or rescue remedy orally and apply them topically. This double strategy works wonders.

Remember, the use of herbal remedies for pain relief is as old as humanity. In modern times, we can wisely and safely add herbal medicines to *The BackCare Blueprint* practices of proactive participation, positive attitudes, proper physical alignment, and breathing techniques to create a well-rounded system of pain relief through purposeful self-care.

It is my greatest wish that the practices and resources provided here finally help you end chronic back pain and begin to enjoy your life again.

THE BACKCARE BLUEPRINT ONLINE COURSE

Personally, I find it more effective to learn new material across a variety of platforms. Perhaps you do, too. To help you integrate the information in this book, I've created an online companion video course for you to follow at home. The videos progress sequentially from the simplest techniques, such as how to "traction your spine", to in-depth guidance of "whole-body" alignment in all the positions you do daily standing, sitting, walking, bending and twisting. I've also recorded several (5-15 minute) practice routines to help you tune up your spine and keep you in a pain-free state. With steady practice and good alignment, you'll be able to say goodbye to pain and hello to joy.

Learn more about the BCB online course here:
https://the-backcare-blueprint.trainercentralsite.com

ADDITIONAL ONLINE RESOURCES

Contact Me:
www.prakasayoga.com/backcareblueprint.cfm

Schedule a free "Get Out of Pain" Consultation:
www.prakasayoga.com/complimentary_consult_schedule.cfm

Work With Me 1:1 Coaching Support:
www.prakasayoga.com/complimentary_consult_schedule.cfm

YouTube Channel: Sacred Being with Lynne Ann Paterson:
www.youtube.com/@PrakasaYoga/featured

Free guided meditations to deepen the mind-body connection and infuse your whole being with vital energy.

LYNNE ANN PATERSON

Lynne has been a student, practitioner, and instructor of yoga since her early twenties. While achieving several professional certifications between 1990-2005, Lynne logged over 10,000 hours of study and practice in the science and art of yoga as a modern healing modality. Her compassion for those in pain, combined with keen observation skills, active intuition, and an acumen for detail makes her a valuable resource for anyone looking for guidance on how to heal themselves. Lynne's ability to distill anatomical jargon into simple language with easy-to-follow instructions makes *The BackCare Blueprint* a timely addition to the existing collection of pain management and back pain relief books.

Lynne suffered with sciatic pain for over a decade, and by necessity, learned to combine structural alignment, physical posture, movement, breathwork and mindset to heal her condition. By changing the patterns that caused her pain, Lynne was able to end the cycle of chronic pain for good. Her aim is to empower people to do the same for themselves.

After working with private clients for over a decade and discovering several common patterns of misalignment, Lynne created a video course to share her method with people who suffer from physical pain. Later, she decided to collect and present that information as *The BackCare Blueprint,* her debut book.

Lynne has a private practice and runs Prakasa Yoga & Wellness Studio in western Massachusetts. You can find more information about her online and in-person programs at www.prakasayoga.com

www.ingramcontent.com/pod-product-compliance
Lightning Source LLC
Chambersburg PA
CBHW052111020426
42335CB00021B/2717

9 7 9 8 9 8 8 0 3 2 7 0 0